Mohamed BELLALI

Focus on electrocution

Mohamed BELLALI

Focus on electrocution

epidemiology and medico-legal aspects

ScienciaScripts

Imprint

Any brand names and product names mentioned in this book are subject to trademark, brand or patent protection and are trademarks or registered trademarks of their respective holders. The use of brand names, product names, common names, trade names, product descriptions etc. even without a particular marking in this work is in no way to be construed to mean that such names may be regarded as unrestricted in respect of trademark and brand protection legislation and could thus be used by anyone.

Cover image: www.ingimage.com

This book is a translation from the original published under ISBN 978-620-6-72135-2.

Publisher:
Sciencia Scripts
is a trademark of
Dodo Books Indian Ocean Ltd. and OmniScriptum S.R.L publishing group

120 High Road, East Finchley, London, N2 9ED, United Kingdom
Str. Armeneasca 28/1, office 1, Chisinau MD-2012, Republic of Moldova, Europe
Printed at: see last page
ISBN: 978-620-8-09048-7

TABLE OF CONTENTS

INTRODUCTION...2

METHODS 3

RESULTS 6

CONCLUSIONS...51

REFERENCES..53

INTRODUCTION

Electricity is the main source of energy, with the United States producing around 4,000 billion kilowatt hours of electricity in 2022 (1). It is used in industry, on construction sites and in domestic homes(2). It is defined as a fluid that propagates through conductive materials(3). Misuse or negligent maintenance of equipment and wiring are the most frequent causes of electrification and, consequently, electrocution(4). Electrification is defined as the passage of an electric current through the human body, with all its pathophysiological manifestations, whereas electrocution is death by electrification. The latter results either from direct contact with a conductive object or indirectly from an electric arc or lightning strike (5).The first fatal occupational accident caused by electrification was in 1879 in France, when a theatre stagehand was struck by a 250 V alternating current (6). And since then, electrical accidents have multiplied, constituting a major health problem because of the significant frequency of the morbidity and mortality they cause. According to the Swiss Federal Inspectorate for Heavy Current Installations ESTI, 572 electrical accidents occurred in Switzerland in 2021, five of which were fatal (7). In the United States, electrification is the 6ème leading cause of death in the workplace, according to the US Bureau of Labor Statistics (3,378 fatalities between 1992 and 2002). In Australia, 162 electrocutions were recorded between 2001 and 2004(8).At national level, the estimated frequency of electrification seems high, but remains imprecise because these accidents do not necessarily result in medical consultation or hospitalisation. On the other hand, statistics relating to electrocutions are feasible because they result in a violent death that poses a medico-legal obstacle to burial and therefore requires a medico-legal autopsy.However, since 2010, only two national studies have investigated the medico-legal aspects of electrocutions : one was carried out in Tunis in 2017 showing a prevalence of 0.6/100,000 inhabitants/year(9) and the other inKairouan in 2020, showing a prevalence of 0.94/100,000 inhabitants/year(10). The lack of recent studies on electrocutions in Tunisia is a real obstacle in terms of public health. Identifying the circumstances in which these accidents occur, their causes, and the shortcomings in routing and treatment is the mainstay of electrification prevention.Death by electrocution also poses a diagnostic problem because electrical marks are not always present, which can mimic a sudden death. Hence the importance of the forensic pathologist's mastery of this subject, especially in the event of death in the workplace, because of the medico-legal and social responsibilities that this would entail.

The aim of our study was to :

- To describe the epidemiological profile and lesion characteristics of the bodies of victims of electrocution in northern Tunisia.

- Recognise the circumstances in which electrocution occurs.

- Suggest areas for improvement in terms of prevention and care for the electrified.

METHODS

1. Type of study :

This was a retrospective descriptive study spread over a four-year period from 1 January 2019 to 31 December 2022 and covering all cases of electrocution autopsied in the Forensic Medicine Department of Charles Nicolle Hospital in Tunis. The service covers 9 of the 11 governorates in northern Tunisia, namely Tunis, Ben Arous, Manouba, Ariana, Beja, Le Kef, Jendouba, Zaghouan and Siliana, representing a general population of 4,282,755 (36% of the Tunisian population) according to the results of the general population and housing census conducted by the National Statistics Institute in 2022(11).

2. Study population :

2.1. Inclusion criteria :

We have included all the bodies autopsied in the forensic medicine department of the Charles Nicolle Hospital whose autopsy concluded that they had been electrocuted.

2.2. Non-inclusion criteria :

We did not include all the cases of corpses autopsied in the forensic medicine department of the Charles Nicolle Hospital in Tunis whose cause of death was other than electrocution. Similarly, cases of Fulguration (electrification by lightning) were not included in our study.

2.3. Exclusion criteria :

We have excluded the cadavers in state of putrefaction state and decomposition.

3. Type of variables and data collection :

The data was collected from the registers of the forensic medicine department and the medico-legal files, each containing a judicial requisition and a copy of the medico-legal autopsy report. The data concerned

3.1. Victim profile :

- Gender.
- Age.

- Family status (single, married, divorced).
- The geographical origin of the victim (urban, rural).
- Level of education (illiterate, primary, secondary, tertiary).

- Socio-economic level (low, medium, high).
- The profession.

- The governorate.
- Pathological history: organic and psychiatric.
- Lifestyle habits (smoking, alcohol, drug abuse).
- Build (light, medium, heavy).

3.2. Circumstances of death :

- The year, month, day and time of occurrence.
- The place of occurrence (at home, in the workplace, on the public highway)
- The characteristics of electric current (high or low voltage).
- Humidity conditions.

- The notion of projection or fall
- Clothing worn at the time of the electrocution.
- The agent involved.

3.3. Care :

- Survival time.

- The delivery method.

- The concept of hospitalisation and the care provided.

3.4. Thanatological findings :

- The electrical brand: type, number, location and size.

- Associated trauma.
- The presumed cause of death.

3.5. The forensic form :

- Accidental :
■ Work-related accident
■ Domestic accident
■ Accident on the public highway
■ Accident following theft of copper

■ Suicidal

■ Criminal

4. Data entry and analysis :

The data collected was entered and analysed using SPSS 23 (Statistics Package for the Social Science). Figures and tables were produced using Microsoft Excel 2013. Qualitative variables were described using percentages and compared using the Pearson Chi-square test or Fisher's exact test for numbers less than five. Quantitative variables were described by means, standard deviations, minimum and maximum values. In all statistical tests, the significance level was set at 0.05.

5. Bibliographic research :

Our bibliography was based on a search for similar scientific studies published in scientific journals, as well as reports from international bodies interested in this subject. We also searched for theses and dissertations defended in the four Tunisian faculties of medicine. Our research was based on the following keywords: electrocution, electrotrauma, autopsy, forensic medicine, cadaver.We searched the following scientific databases: Embase (Elsevier), Med line (PubMed), Science direct, Google scholar and Cochrane Library.

6. Ethical aspects and conflicts of interest :

The data collected was used for purely scientific purposes. Anonymity has been respected, and victims' names have been replaced by numbers. We declare that we have no conflict of interest in relation to this work.

RESULTS

At the end of this study, we collated 9021 cases of death, 126 of which were victims of electrocution and which underwent a medico-legal autopsy at the forensic medicine department of Charles Nicolle Hospital in Tunis, recorded between 1er January 2019 and 31 December 2022 (Figure 1).

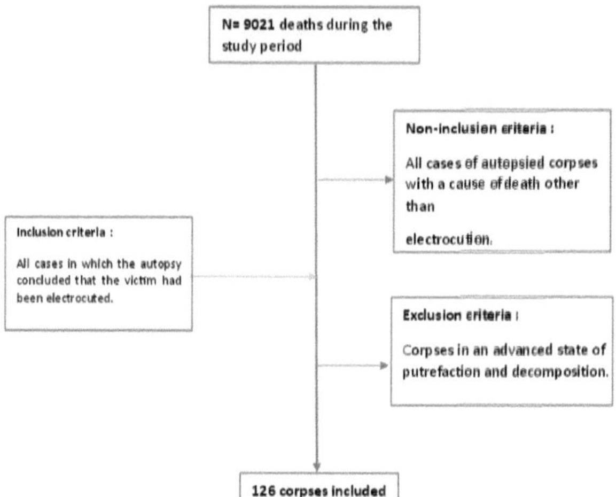

Figure 1: Flow chart for selecting the study sample

1. Description of the population :

1.1. Prevalence of electrocution compared with the general population

During the period of our study, the average population of our study region (northern Tunisia excluding Bizerte and Nabeul) was estimated at 4,245,642(11). The number of victims of electrocution autopsied in our department was 126, i.e. an average of 31.5 cases per year. This represented an average rate of 0.74/100,000 inhabitants. (Table 1)

Table I: Prevalence of electrocution in the general population

Année	Number	Population	Rates electrocution /per 100,000 inhabitants
2019	31	4 214 750	0,74
2020	26	4 242 485	0,61
2021	41	4 259 963	0,96
2022	28	4 282 755	0,65
Average total	31,5	4 249 988	0,74

1.2. Prevalence of electrocutions in relation to the department's activity :

Electrocutions represented an average of 1.4% of our department's thanatological activity over the 4 years of the study, from 2019 to 2022. We recorded a peak of 1.8% in 2021. (Table 2)

Table II: Prevalence of electrocution cases in relation to department activity

Année	Nombre d'électrocution	Nombre total d'autopsie	Pourcentage d'électrocution (%)
2019	31	2379	1,3
2020	26	2121	1,2
2021	41	2316	1,8
2022	28	2205	1,3
Total	126	9021	1,4

2. Victim profile :

2.1. Breakdown by age :

The average age of those electrocuted was 39.68 years, with extremes ranging from 8 months to 77 years. The age distribution showed that 47.6 % of cases were aged between 18 and 39. Seven cases of electrocution in children (under 18 years of age) were recorded (5.6%). We recorded 15 victims aged over 60, i.e. 11.9% of the total. Males predominated in all age groups (Figure 2).

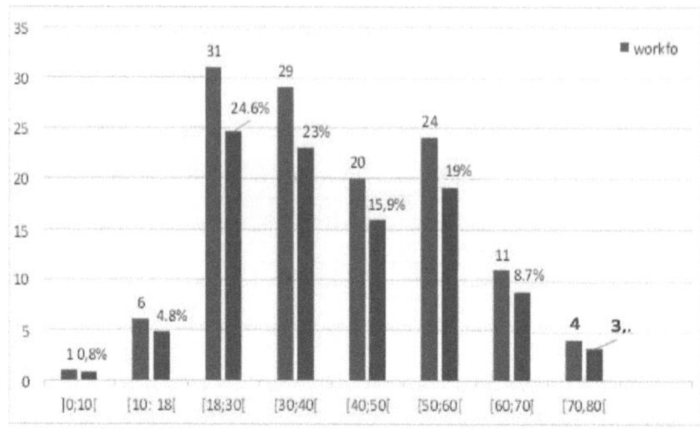

Figure 2: Breakdown by age group

2.2. Breakdown by gender :

The breakdown of victims by sex showed that they were predominantly male, with a percentage of 90% and a sex ratio (M/F) of 9.5 (Figure 3).

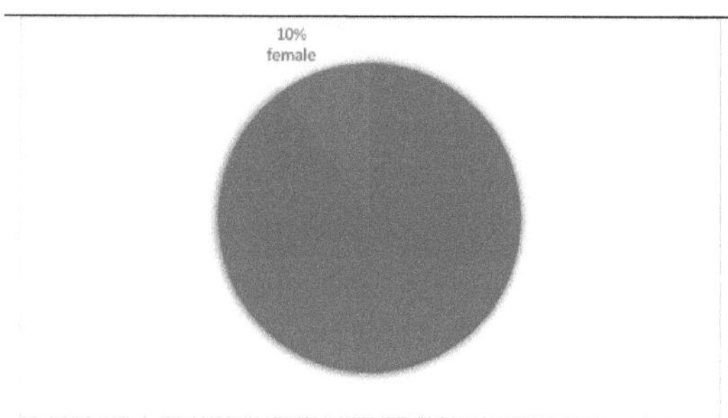

Figure 3: Breakdown by gender

2.3. Breakdown by age and gender :

The age range 18 to 39 was predominant for both sexes: 63 men (55.3%) and 6 women (50%). There were no cases of electrocution among women under the age of 18. The age group least affected was after 60 for male victims (10.5%). We did not find a significant relationship between age and gender (p=0.5). (Figure 4).

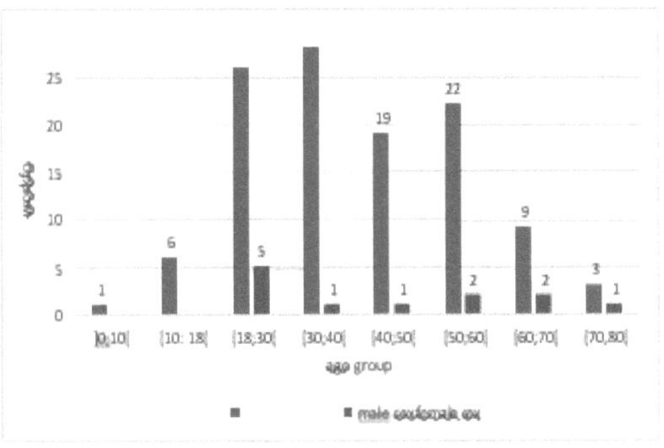

Figure 4: Breakdown by age group and gender

2.4. Breakdown by geographical origin :

71.4% of the victims (90 cases) were of urban origin and 28.6% (36 cases) of rural origin. were of rural origin. (Figure 5)

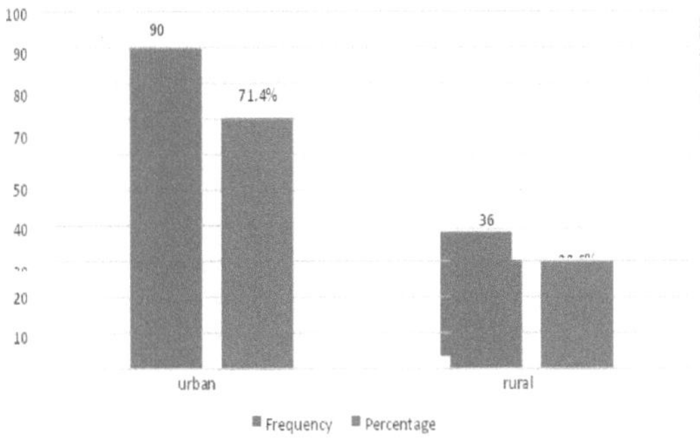

Figure 5: Breakdown by geographical origin

2.5. Breakdown by family status :

53.2% of the victims were married (67 cases) and 43.7% were single. Four victims were divorced. (Table 3)

Table III: Breakdown by family status

Family status	Workforce	Percentage (%)
Single	55	43,7
Married	67	53,2
Divorced	4	3,2
total	126	100

2.6. Breakdown by victim's occupation :

Day labourers represented the occupational category most affected, with a percentage of 61.1%. Factory workers accounted for only 1.6%. Housewives, children and unemployed young people fell into the no occupation category. (Table 4)

Table IV: Breakdown by profession

	Frequency	Percentage (%)
Worker	77	61 ,1
Factory worker	2	1,6
Electrical installation	8	6,3
Retired	6	4,8
No profession	27	21,4
Undetermined	6	4,8
total	126	100

2.7. Breakdown by governorate :

In our series of studies, there was a clear predominance of cases occurring in the governorates of Greater Tunis (80.1%). The lowest frequency of victims (2.4%) was recorded in Siliana (Figure 6).

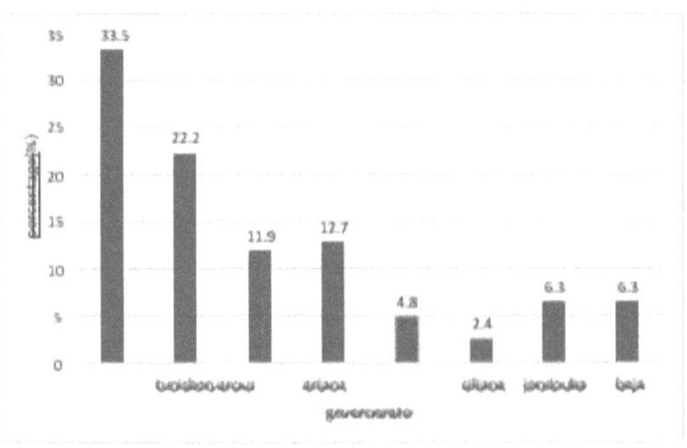

Figure 6: Breakdown by governorate

2.8. Breakdown by level of education :

67.5% of victims had a primary education, while 2.4% had a secondary education. of cases had a higher level of education. (Table 5)

Table V: Breakdown by educational level

	Frequency	Percentage (%)
Illiterate	3	2,4
Primary	85	67,5
Secondary	35	27,8
Superior	3	2,4
Total	126	100

2.9. Breakdown by socio-economic level :

66.7% of victims had an average socio-economic level, 28.6% had a low level and only 4.8% of cases had a high level (Figure 7).

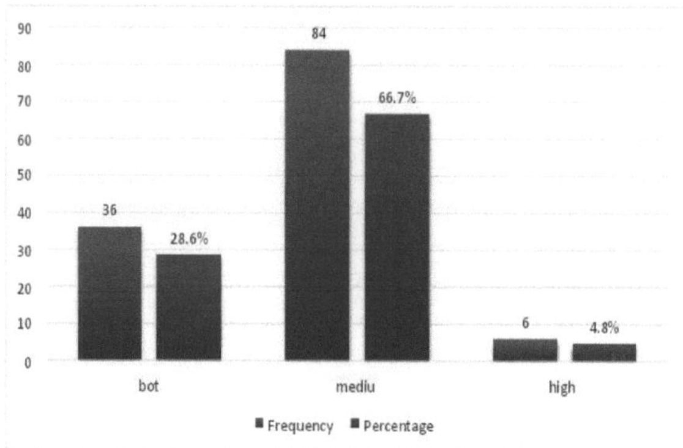

Figure 7: Socio-economic level

2.10. Breakdown by antecedents :

80.1% of the victims had no medical or surgical history. Only two victims (1.6%) had psychiatric disorders. With regard to other antecedents, one victim had isolated heart disease, only one victim was hypertensive, 3 victims were diabetic (2.4%) and one victim had a heart condition.12 victims had a history of surgery (9.5%). Six victims had suffered from heart disease associated with other chronic conditions (4.8%). (Figure 8)

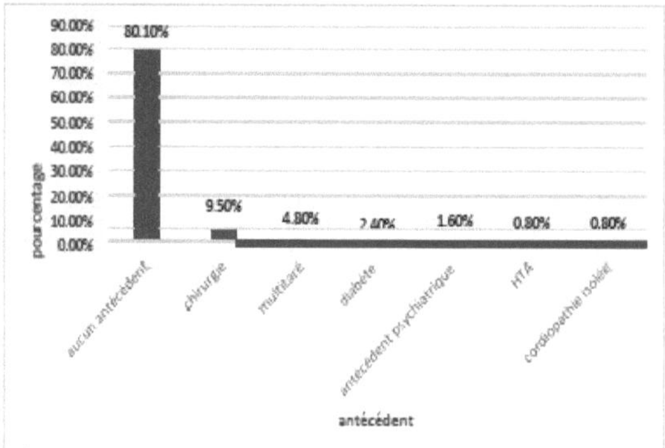

Figure 8: Breakdown by antecedents

2.11. Breakdown by lifestyle :

61.2% of the victims had no addiction problems. 19% were smokers only. 19% were smokers and alcoholics. Only one victim was a smoker, alcoholic and drug addict (Figure 9).

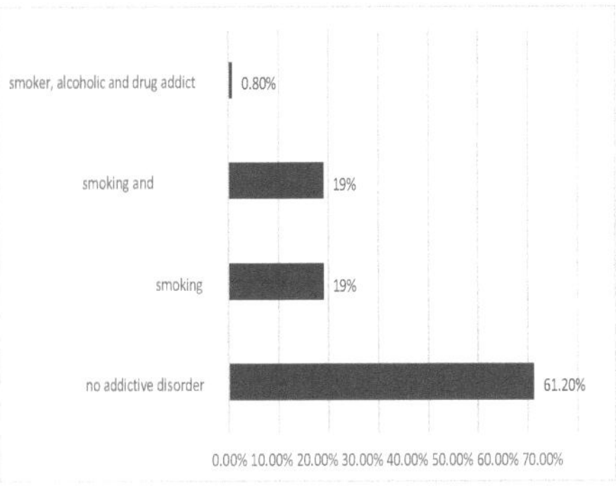

Figure 9: Breakdown by lifestyle habits

2.12. Breakdown by build :

72.2% of victims were of average build. Victims of heavy build accounted for 18.3% and those of light build for 9.5%. (Figure 10).

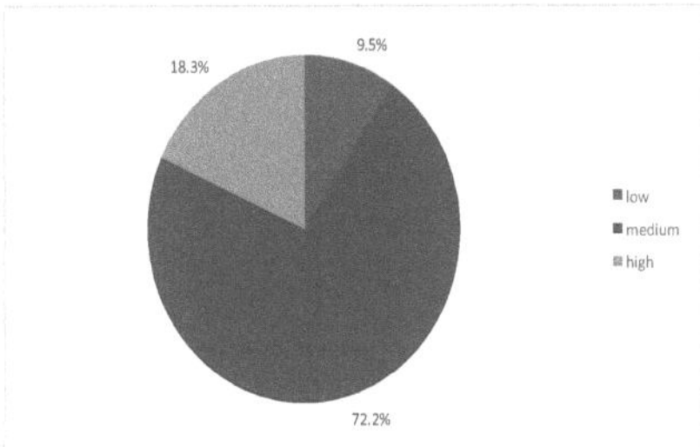

Figure 10: Breakdown by build

3. Circumstances of electrocution :

3.1. Distribution of victims over time :

3.1.1. Breakdown by month :

Electrocution was most frequent in July and August, with a percentage of 17.5% each, followed by September with a percentage of 15.9%. The rest of the months had lower percentages ranging from 3.2% to 8.7% (Figure 11).

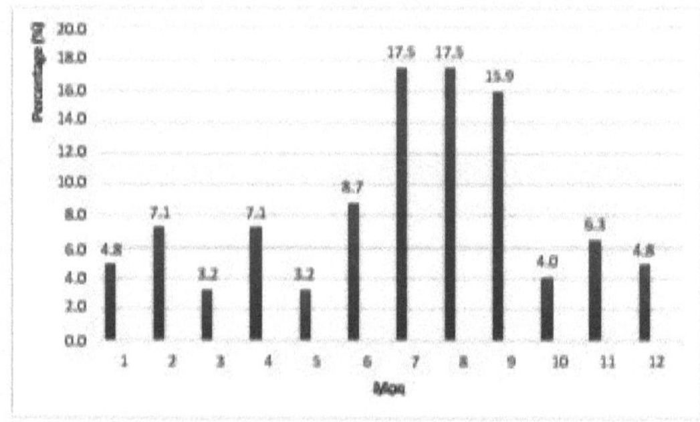

Figure 11: Breakdown by month

3.1.2. Breakdown by season :

44% of electrocutions occurred in the summer, followed by autumn (25%) and winter (17%). The lowest frequency of electrocutions occurred in spring (14%). (Figure 12).

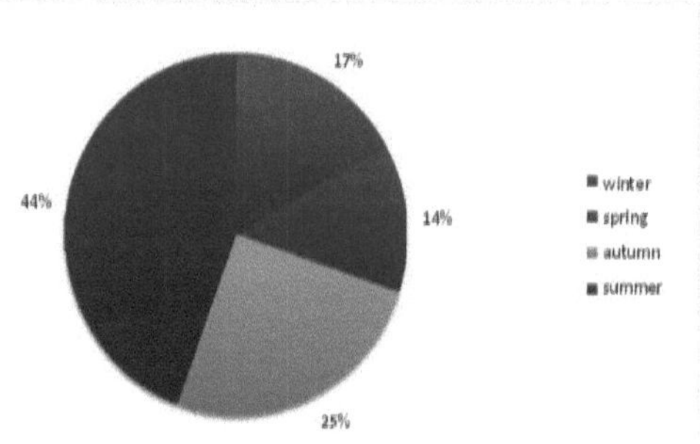

Figure 12: Breakdown by season

3.1.3. Breakdown by day of the week :

Two peaks in frequency were observed on Saturdays and Wednesdays, with 19% and 18.3% respectively. On the other days, the frequency of electrocution varied between 10.3% and 14.3% (Figure 13).

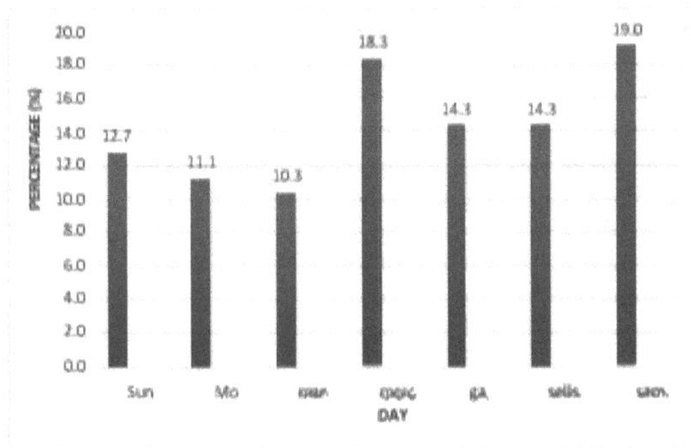

Figure 13: Breakdown by day of the week

3.1.4. Breakdown by time of death :

45.2% of electrocutions occurred in the afternoon, between 12pm and 6pm. The time period least affected was midnight to six in the morning, with a percentage of 2.4% (Figure14).

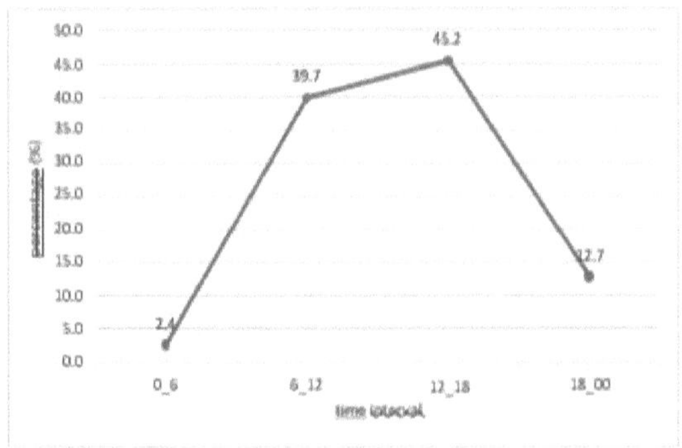

Figure 14: Breakdown by time of occurrence

3.2. Breakdown by place of death :

46.8% of electrocutions occurred in the home, 34.1% in the workplace and only 19% on public roads (Figure 15).

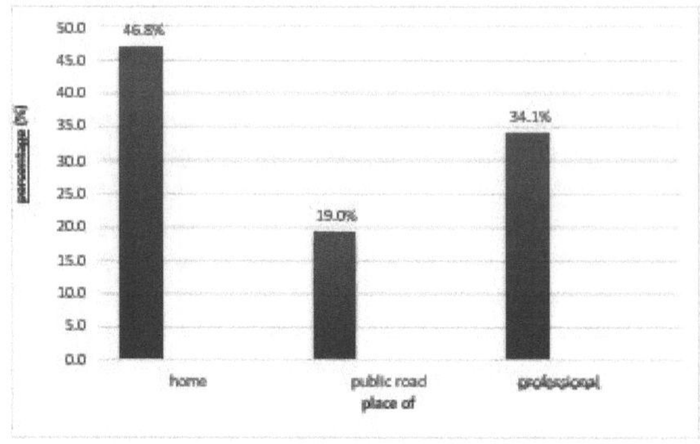

Figure 15: Breakdown by place of occurrence

3.3. Distribution according to humidity conditions :

71.4% of electrocutions occurred in dry conditions and 28.6% in wet conditions (Figure 16).

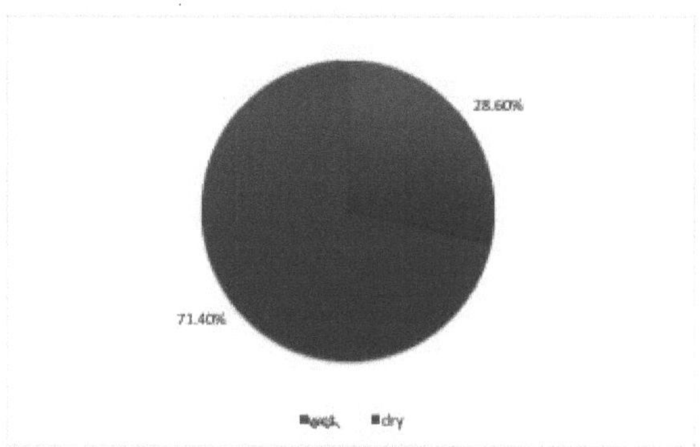

Figure 16: Breakdown by environment

3.4. Distribution according to the nature of the electric current :

High voltage current was responsible for 52.5% of electrocutions (66 cases), while low voltage was involved in 47.6%. (Figure 17).

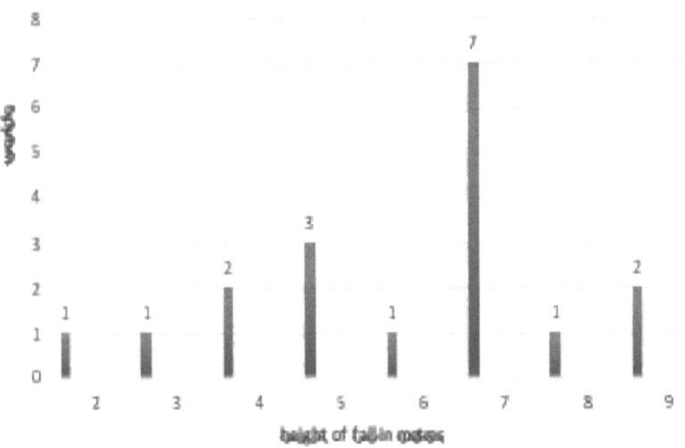

Figure 18: Breakdown by height of fall

3.6. Breakdown by agent involved :

The majority of electrocutions were caused by a bare cable (64.3%). 31 victims were electrocuted by faulty electrical equipment (24.6%). The remaining victims were electrocuted by contact with an electrical socket (Figure 19).

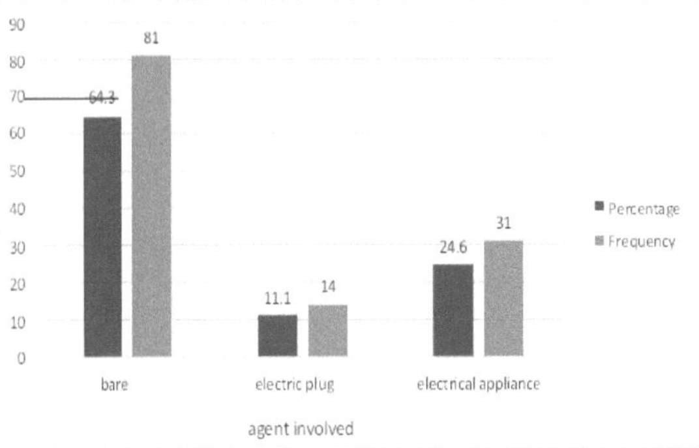

Figure 19: Breakdown by agent involved

3.7. Breakdown by gender and location of electrocution :

All the women had been electrocuted at home. However, all the electrocutions that occurred on the public highway and in the workplace involved exclusively male victims. We found a significant relationship between the gender of the victim and the place of electrocution (p = 0.001). (Figure 20).

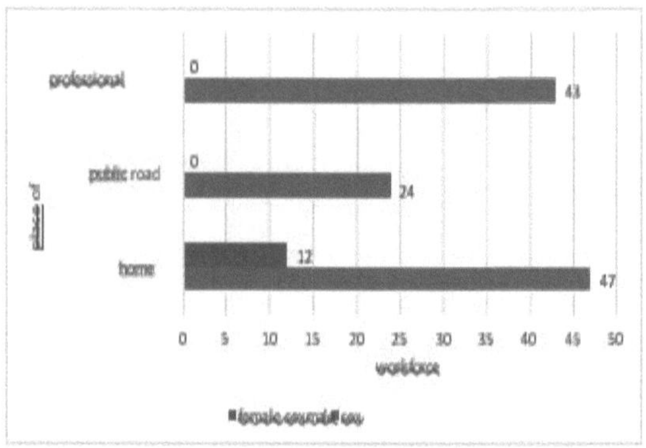

Figure 20: Breakdown by gender and place of occurrence

3.8. Distribution according to age and place of electrocution :

The extreme age groups (<10 years and >69 years) were all electrocuted at home. Occupational electrocutions began to appear from the age of 18 and their frequency increased progressively with age, reaching a maximum of 11 occupational electrocutions between the ages of 50 and 59. Street electrocutions predominated among young people aged between 20 and 39, with a total of 16 cases (66.7%). We found a significant relationship between age and the place where the electrocution occurred (p=0.01). (Figure 21).

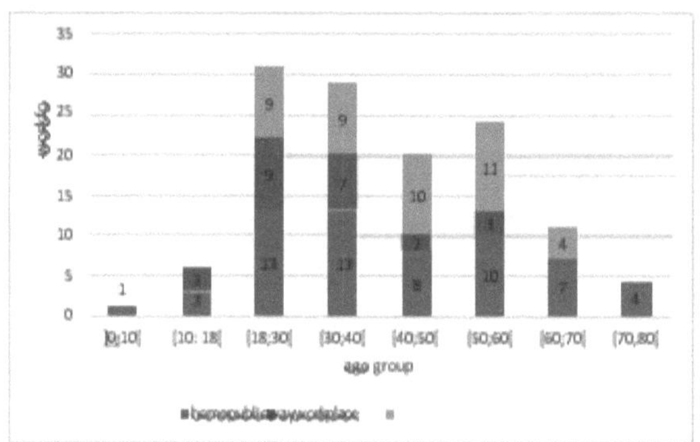

Figure 21 : Breakdown by age and place of occurrence

3.9. Breakdown by occupation and place of occurrence :

Fatal occupational electrical injuries were predominant among manual workers (81.4%). The majority of electrical installation workers were electrocuted in the workplace (87.5%). Among non-occupational victims, electrocution occurred more frequently at home (66.7%). We found a significant relationship between occupation and place of electrocution (p= 0.000014). (Figure 22).

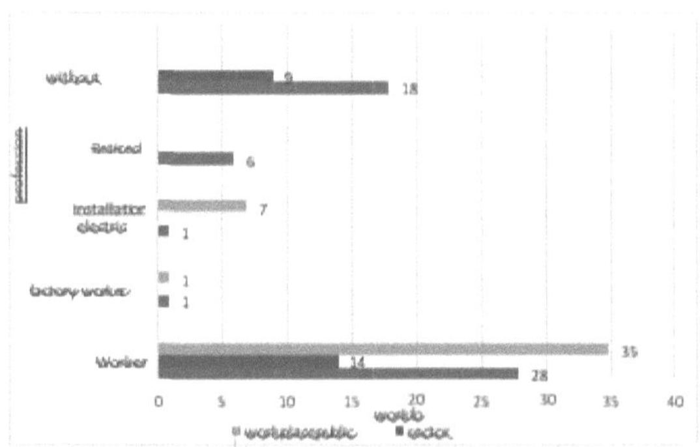

Figure 22: Breakdown by occupation and place of occurrence

3.10. Breakdown by type of electric current and place of electrocution :

Low-voltage electrocutions occurred in the home in 68.3% of cases. 60.5% of electrocutions that occurred in the workplace were caused by a high-voltage current. We found a significant relationship between the type of current and the location of the electrocution (p=0.00001) (Table 6).

Table VI: Breakdown by electric current and place of occurrence

	Home	Public roads	Professional environment
High voltage current	18	22	26
Low voltage current	41	2	17
Total	59	24	43

3.11. Distribution according to the agent involved and the location of the electrocution :

Bare cables were the cause of death in all cases of electrocution on the public highway. The majority of fatal electrical injuries involving plugs occurred in the home (92.9%). We found a significant relationship between the agent involved and the place of electrocution p=0.000015) (Figure 23).

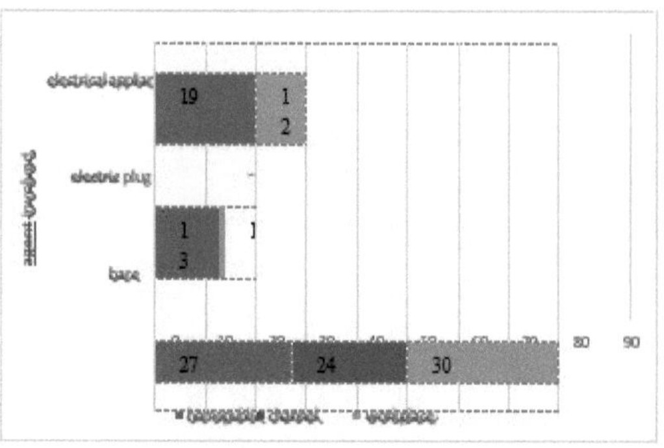

Figure 23: Breakdown by causal agent and place of occurrence

The relationships between the location of the electrocution and the various parameters (gender, occupation, nature of the current and causal agent) and the statistical values are summarised in table 7.

Table VII: Relationship between location of electrocution and various parameters

	Lieu de l'électrocution			Valeur de P
	Travail	Domicile	Voie publique	
Genre				
Homme	43	47	24	0,001
Femme	0	12	0	
Profession				
Ouvrier	35	28	14	
Installation électrique	7	1	0	
Sans profession	0	18	9	0,000014
Retraité	0	6	0	
Travailleur d'usine	1	1	0	
Nature du courant				
Haute tension	26	18	22	0,00001
Basse tension	17	41	2	
L'agent causal				
Câble nu	30	27	24	
Appareil défectueux	12	19	0	0,000015
Prise électrique	13	1	0	

3.12. Breakdown by agent involved and gender :

Almost all the victims electrocuted by bare cables were men (98.8%). Women were electrocuted by an electrical socket in 58.3% of cases. The agent involved varied significantly according to gender (p<0.00001) (Figure 24).

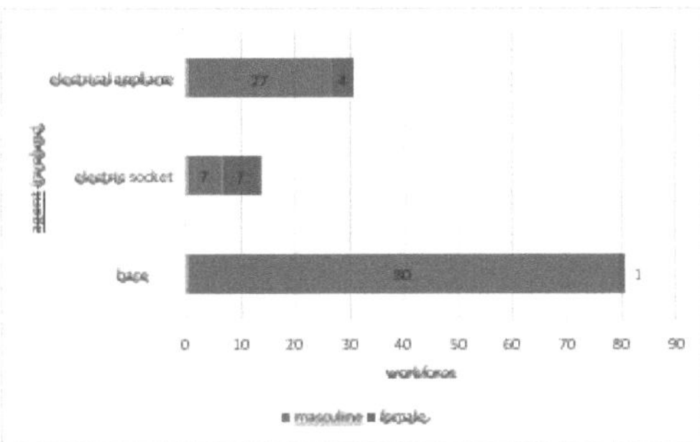

Figure 24: Breakdown by agent involved and gender

3.13. Breakdown by agent and age group :

Electrocution by a bare cable was frequently observed in all age groups except the oldest. The only victim under the age of 10 was electrocuted by contact with an electrical socket. For the 4 victims aged over 69, the causal agent of the electrocution was a faulty electrical appliance in 3 cases and an electrical socket in only one case. We did not find a significant relationship between the causal agent and age (p=0.08). (Figure 25)

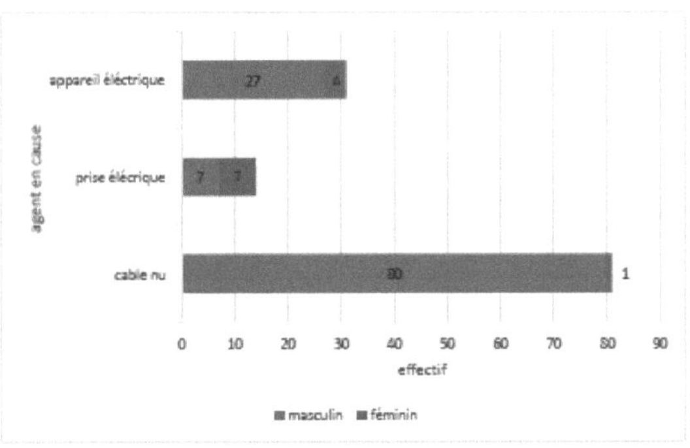

Figure 25 : Breakdown by agent involved and age

4.Support :

4.1. Breakdown by survival time :

79.4% of victims died within the first 24 hours following electrocution (100 victims). Only 26 victims survived beyond 24 hours (20.6%) (Figure26).

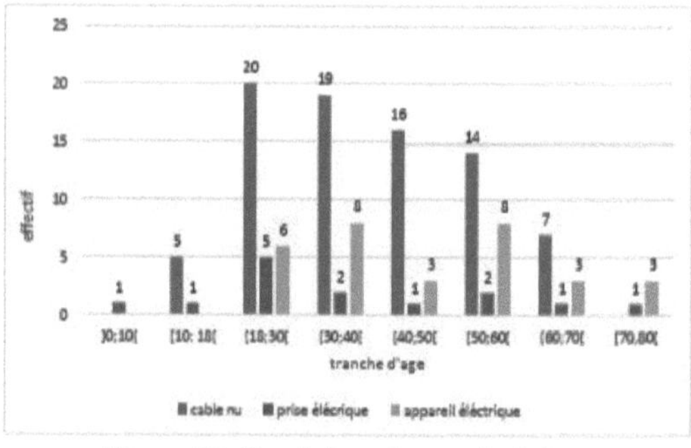

Figure 26: Breakdown by survival time

4.2. Breakdown by delivery mode :

No victims were transported by the emergency medical service. (SAMU). Only one victim was transported by a non ambulance (type B). The majority of victims were transported by the civil protection (83.3%). The remaining victims (15.9%) were transported by their own means. (Table 8).

Table VIII: Breakdown by mode of transport

	Workforce	Percentage
Clean average	20	15,9%
Civil protection	105	83,3%
Ambulance type B	1	0,8%
SAMU	0	0%
TOTAL	126	100%

4.3. Breakdown by type of care :

62.7% of the victims had died at the scene and had not received any medical treatment (79 cases). Only one victim had received treatment at the scene. The rest of the victims (46 cases) had received hospital treatment (Table 9).

Table IX: Breakdown by type of care provided

	Workforce	Percentage
No care	79	62,7%
On-site care	1	0,8%
Hospital care	46	36,5%
Total	126	100%

4.4. Breakdown by type of electric current and survival time :

93.3% of victims electrocuted by a low-voltage current died within the first 24 hours (56 cases). 84.6% of victims who survived beyond 24 hours had been electrocuted with a high-voltage current (n=22). Survival time varied significantly according to the type of electric current (p=0.0003). (Table 10)

Table X: Breakdown by type of current and survival time

	High voltage	Low voltage	Total
Survival less than 24 hours	44	56	100
Survival over 24 hours	22	4	26
Total	66	60	126

4.5. Distribution according to care administered and survival time :

56.5% of victims who had received medical attention in hospital had survived beyond 24 hours (n=26). All victims who did not receive medical care died within the first 24 hours (n=79). Survival time varied significantly with the care administered (p<0.000001). (Table 11)

Table XI: Distribution according to care provided and survival time

	No care	Care on place	Care for the hospital	Total
Survival less than 24 hours	79	1	20	100
Survival over 24 hours	0	0	26	26
Total	79	1	46	126

4.6. **Distribution according to survival time and humidity :**

94.4% of victims electrocuted in a wet environment had survived less than 24 hours (34 cases). 92.3% of victims surviving beyond 24 hours were electrocuted in a dry environment (24 cases). Survival time varied significantly with humidity (p=0.005). (Figure 27)

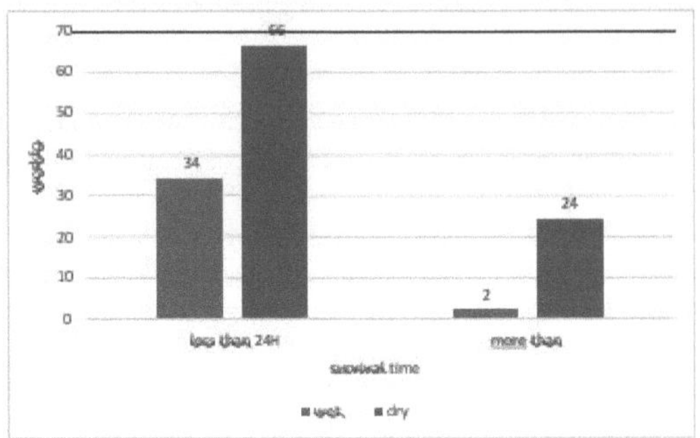

Figure 27: Distribution according to survival time and humidity

4.7. **Breakdown by survival time and agent involved :**

All the victims electrocuted by a faulty electrical appliance died within the first 24 hours (31 cases). Only one victim electrocuted by contact with an electrical socket survived beyond 24 hours. 96.2% of victims who survived beyond 24 hours were electrocuted by a bare cable (25 cases). Survival time varied significantly according to the causal agent (p=0.001). (Table 12)

Table XII: Breakdown by survival time and causative agent

	Bare cable	Electrical socket	Electrical appliance	Total
Survival less than 24 hours	56	13	31	100
Survival over 24 hours	25	1	0	26
Total	81	14	31	126

The relationships between survival time and the various parameters (type of current, treatment administered, humidity condition and causal agent) and statistical values are summarised in Table 13.

Table XIII: Distribution according to survival time and different parameters

	Délai de survie		Valeur de p
	Moins de 24h	Plus de 24h	
Nature du courant			
Haute tension	44	22	p=0,0003
Basse tension	56	4	
Soins administrés			
Pas de soin	79	0	
Soins sur place	1	0	p<0,000001
Soins à l'hôpital	20	26	
Agent en cause			
Câble nu	56	25	
Appareil électrique	31	0	p=0,001
Prise électrique	13	1	
Condition d'humidité			
Sec	66	24	p=0.005
Humide	34	2	

1. Thanatological findings :

1.1. Breakdown by electrical brand :

1.1.1. Breakdown of electrical brands by type :

90 victims had electrical marks (71.4%). These electrical marks were an entry door alone in 43 victims (34.1%), an exit door alone in 10 victims (7.9%). A combination of an entry and exit door was observed in 37 victims (29.4%). (Table 14)

Table XIV: Breakdown of electrical brands by type

	Workforce	Percentage
No marks	36	28,6%
Entrance door only	43	34,1%
Exit door only	10	7,9%
Entrance + exit door	37	29,4%
Total	126	100%

1.1.2. **Breakdown by number of electrical brands :**

The average number of electrical brands was 2.74, with a maximum of 10 and a minimum of one. Figure 27 shows the distribution of cases according to the number of electrical brands.

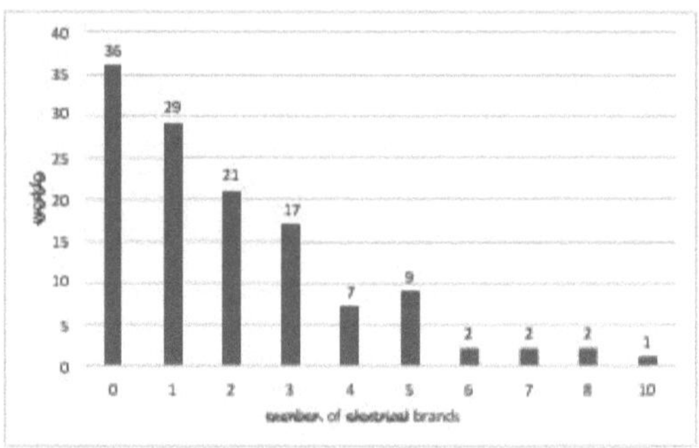

Figure 28: Breakdown by number of electrical brands

1.1.3. **Breakdown of electrical brands by location :**

The majority of electrical marks were found on both upper limbs (65.8%), with a predominance on the left upper limb (35.5%). 32.2% had electrical marks on both lower limbs, predominantly on the right lower limb (18.7%). We did not observe any electrical marks on the victims' heads or necks. (Table 15)

Table XV: Breakdown of electrical brands by location

Electrical brand	Workforce	Percentage
Left upper limb	55	35,5%
Right upper limb	47	30,3%
Right lower limb	29	18,7%
Lower left limb	21	13,5%
Thorax	2	1,3%
Abdomen	1	0,7%
Head and neck	0	0%
TOTAL	155	100%

1.1.4. **Breakdown by location of front door :**

The left upper limb alone was the site of the portal of entry in 39 victims, followed by the right upper limb (29 cases). Both upper limbs had an entry site in 10 cases. Only two victims had other entry sites. One was in the left lower limb and the other in the thorax (Figure 28).

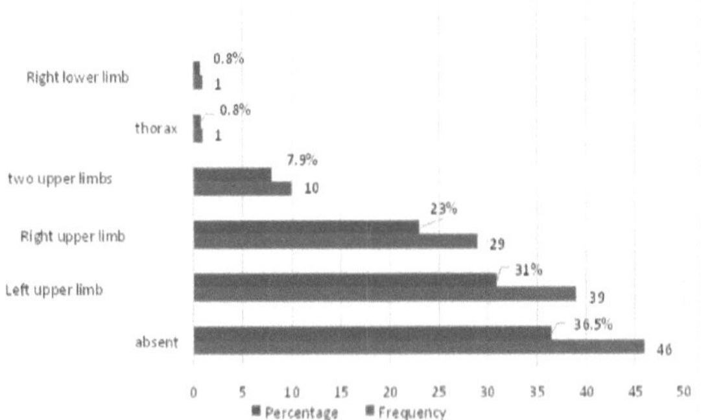

Figure 28: Breakdown by gateway location

1.1.5. **Breakdown by exit door location :**

The right lower limb was the most frequent site of entry (28 cases), followed by the left lower limb (19 cases). (Figure 29).

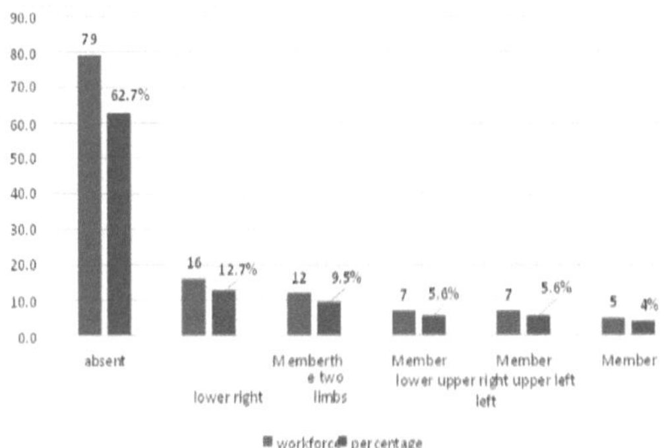

Figure 29: Breakdown by exit door location

1.1.6. Breakdown by electrical brand size :

47.8% of electrical marks were between one and five centimetres in size. Large electrical marks (greater than five centimetres) were present in 12.2% of cases. Sub-centimetre electrical marks were present in 40% of cases. (Figure 30)

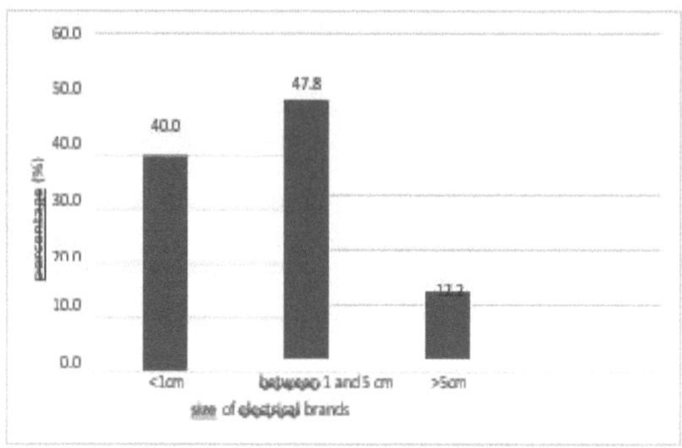

Figure 30: Distribution according to the exit door seat

1.2. Distribution according to the presence or absence of an asphyxia syndrome :

The asphyxia syndrome was present in 75.4% of victims. It was represented by pulmonary oedema in 75.4% of victims, cerebral oedema in 73% and poly-visceral congestion in 66.7%. (Figure 31)

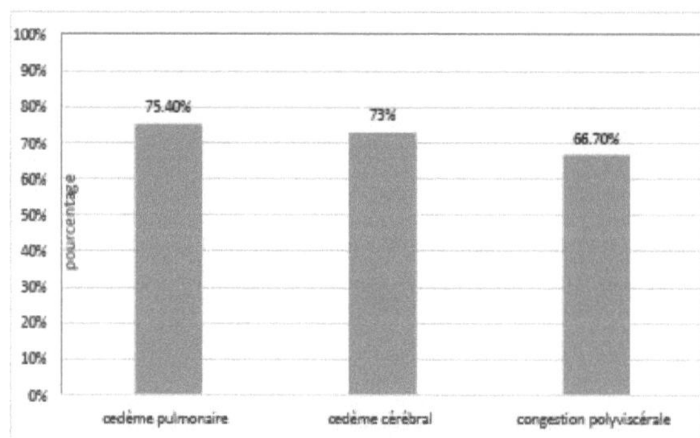

Figure 31: Breakdown by autopsy signs of asphyxia syndrome

1.3. Distribution according to injuries associated with electrocution :

Traumatic injuries were observed in 44 victims (34.9%). 35 victims had head injuries. 21 victims had thoracic trauma. Abdominal trauma was observed in 9 victims. Four victims had pelvic trauma and six victims had peripheral trauma. Polytrauma was observed in 11 cases. (Table 16)

Table XVI: Breakdown by associated trauma

	Workforce	Percentage
Head trauma	35	27,8%
Scalp lesion	35	27,8%
Subdural haematoma	11	8,7%
Intracerebral haematoma	5	4%
Meningeal haemorrhage	8	6,3%
Fracture of the skull bones	8	6,3%
Thoracic trauma	21	16,7%
Fractured ribs	18	14,3%
Lung lesions	6	4,8%
Cardiac lesions	2	1,6%
Abdominal trauma	9	7,1%
Liver damage	8	6,4%
Splenic lesions	1	0,8%
Kidney damage	7	5,6%
Pancreatic lesions	2	1,6%
Trauma to the pelvis	4	3,2%
Peripheral trauma	6	4,8%
Trauma to the spine	6	4,8%
polytrauma	11	8,7%

1.4. Breakdown by burns and skin lesions :

43 victims had burns (34.1%). Of these, 14 cases had second-degree burns (32.6% of burns) and 29 cases had third-degree burns (67.4% of burns). 4.8% of victims had "crocodile skin" type skin lesions (6 cases). 7.1% of victims had charring lesions (9 cases). 3.2% of victims had vascular arborisation (4 cases).

1.5. Additional post-mortem examinations :

1.5.1. Toxicological report :

A toxicology sample was taken in 45.2% of cases (57 victims). Only one victim had a positive toxicology report with a blood alcohol level of 0.69g/l. Toxicology results were negative in 8.7% of cases, and the remaining samples (35.7%) were not recovered.

1.5.2. Anatomopathological examination :

An anatomopathological examination was carried out in 9.5% of cases (12 victims). Only two results were recovered. The first involved a skin fragment and showed epidermal changes consistent with a burn. The second sample concerned organ fragments and showed, in the heart: a focal dense eosinophilic appearance of myocardial cells with no neutrophils, indicating acute cellular suffering; in the lungs: recent focal alveolar haemorrhage with no other abnormalities apart from moderate non-inflammatory oedema. The congestive brain, cerebellum, trunk, pancreatic, renal and splenic tissues were without significant abnormalities.

1.6. Breakdown by terminal mechanism of death :

The final cause of death was isolated electrocution in 68.3% of cases. In 19.8% of cases, death was secondary to septic shock complicating extensive, deep and superinfected electrical burns in all victims who were hospitalised. In 11.9% of cases, the final cause of death was the association between electrocution and serious trauma.

1.7. Breakdown by medico-legal form :

The accidental form was the most frequent (97.6% of cases). The forensic form was suicidal in only three victims. We did not record any homicides secondary to electrocution. (Figure 32).

Figure 32: Breakdown by medico-legal form

The accidental form was divided into four types: 47.6% of victims were electrocuted following a domestic accident, 34.1% following an accident at work, 14.3% following a road traffic accident and 1.6% of cases were electrocuted during a copper theft. (Figure 33).

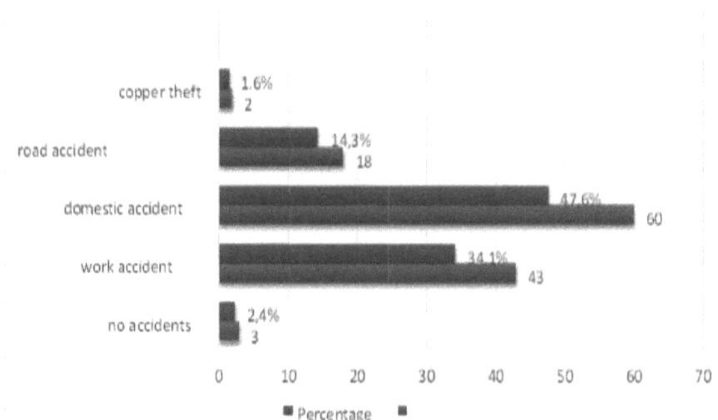

Figure 33: Breakdown by type of accident

1.8. Breakdown by type of current and associated trauma

High-voltage current was responsible for 61.4% of the injuries associated with electrocution (27 cases). 38.6% of the injuries observed were caused by electrocution with a low-voltage current. The presence or absence of trauma did not vary significantly according to the type of electric current (p=0.19). (Figure 34)

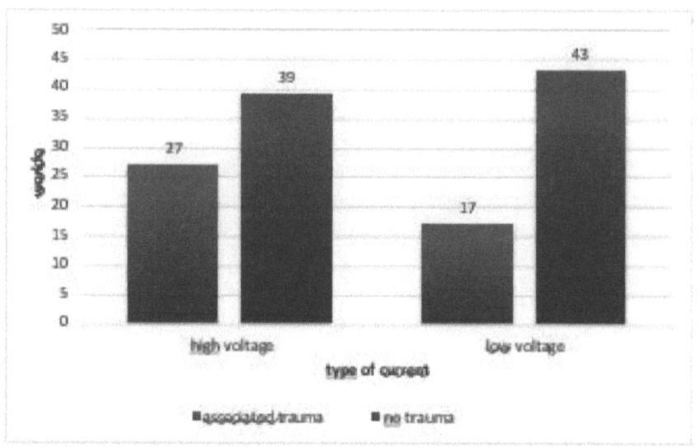

Figure 34: Breakdown by type of current and associated trauma

1.9. Breakdown by type of current and electrical brand :

65.2% of victims electrocuted by a high voltage current had electrical marks (43 cases). Electrical marks were present in 71.7% of victims of electrocution by a low-voltage current. The presence or absence of electrical marks did not vary significantly according to the type of electric current (p=0.43). (Figure 35)

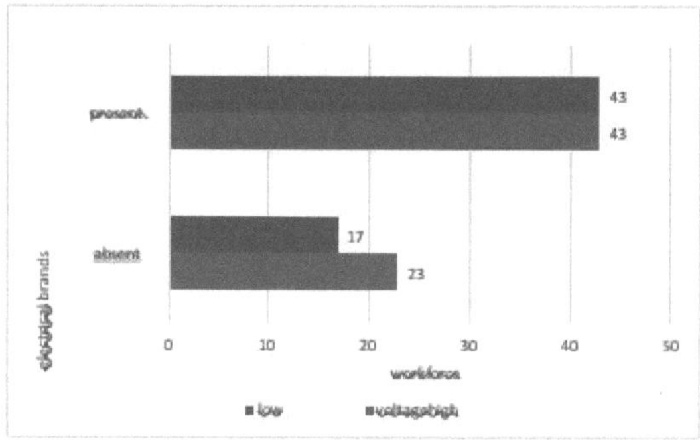

Figure 35: Breakdown by type of current and electrical brand

1.10. Breakdown by type of current and size of electrical brand :

81.8% of victims with extensive electrical marks (>5cm) had been electrocuted by a high-voltage current (9 cases). However, 66.7% of victims with sub-centimetre electrical marks had been electrocuted by a low-voltage current (24 cases). The size of the electrical marks varied significantly according to the type of current (p=0.02) (Figure 36).

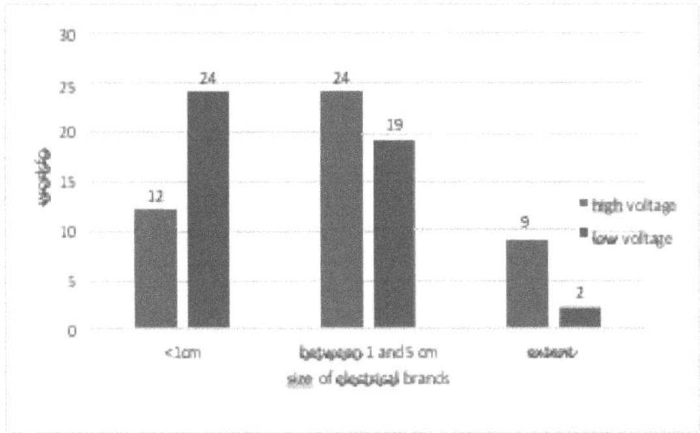

Figure 36: Breakdown by type of current and brand size

Distribution according to the nature of the current and the terminal mechanism of death : 88% of victims who died from septic shock secondary to extensive electrical burns (22 cases) and 86.7% of victims who died from electrocution associated with serious trauma (13 cases) had been electrocuted by a high-voltage current. 91.7% of victims electrocuted by a low-voltage current (55 cases) died from isolated electrocution. The mechanism of death varied significantly according to the nature of the electric current (p=0.00005). (Figure 37)

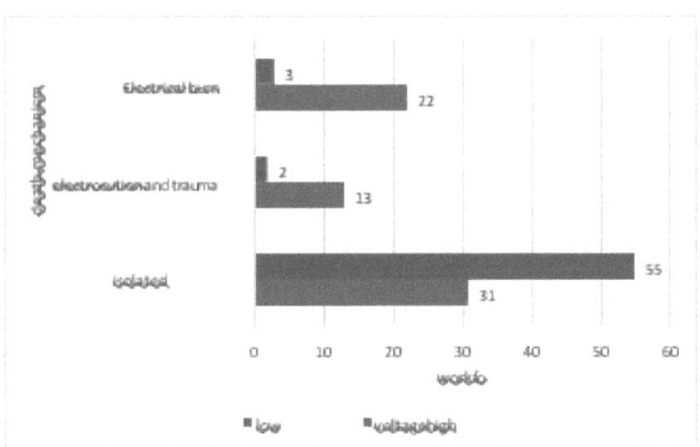

Figure 37: Breakdown by type of current and fatal mechanism

1.11. Breakdown by type of current and medico-legal form :

The three cases of suicide that we recorded were electrocuted by a high-voltage current. We did not find a significant relationship between the nature of the current and the forensic form (p=0.24). (Figure 38)

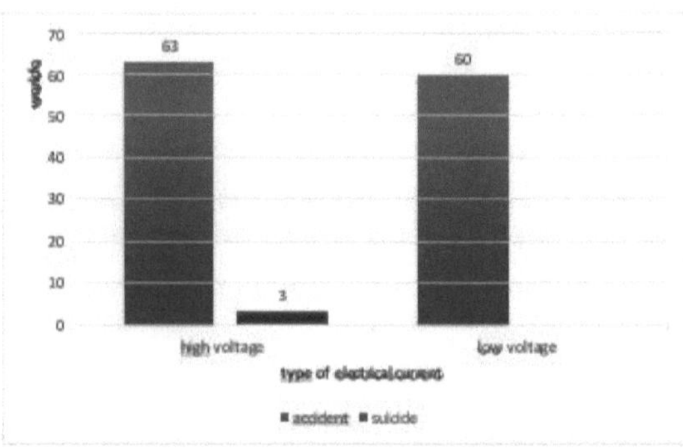

Figure 38: Breakdown by type of current and forensic form

88.9% of victims of a road traffic accident were electrocuted by a high voltage current (16 cases). 68.3% of victims of domestic accidents were electrocuted by low-voltage current (41 cases). Contact with a high-voltage current was the cause of 60.5% of deaths in accidents at work. The two cases of electrocution following the theft of copper were caused by high-voltage current. We found a significant relationship between the nature of the current and the type of accident (p=0.000008). (Figure 39).

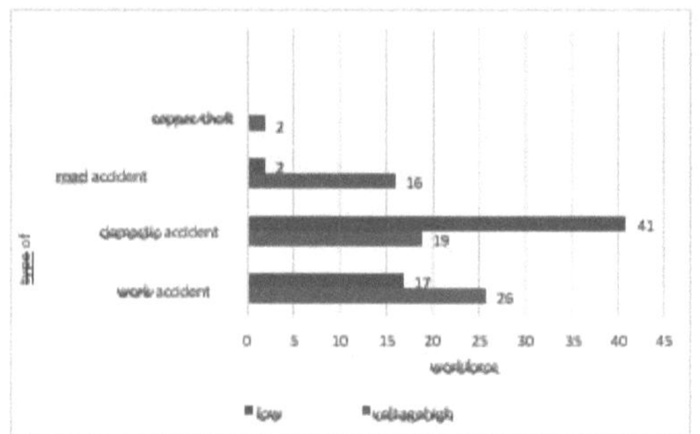

Figure 39: Breakdown by type of current and type of accident

Our study focused on deaths by electrocution autopsied in the forensic medicine department of Charles Nicole Hospital in Tunis over a four-year period from 1er January 2019 to 31 December 2022. Our sample consisted of 126 cases. Electrocution was observed more frequently in men than in women, with a sex ratio equal to 9.5. The mean age was 39.68 years, with extremes of 8 months and 77 years. The age group most affected was between 18 and 39 (47.6%). 61.1% of those electrocuted were blue-collar workers.Electrocutions occurred more frequently in the afternoon from 12pm to 6pm (45.2%), on Saturdays (19%), during the summer season (44%) and in Greater Tunis (80.1%): 47.6% domestic accidents, 34.1% accidents at work, 14.3% road accidents and 1.6% of cases were electrocuted following an attempt to steal copper. High voltage current was responsible for 52.5% of electrocutions. In 64.3% of cases, the causal agent was a bare cable. The majority of victims died within the first 24 hours (79.4%). None of the victims were transported by ambulance. 62.7% of victims died at the scene and did not receive any medical treatment.

1. Interest and limitations of the study :

The aim of this study was to establish a specific epidemiological profile by highlighting the prevalence of work-related electrical accidents among young people (1er work-related accidents at the age of 18), which could be a determining factor in the implementation of targeted prevention measures.

Our study presented limitations linked to the retrospective nature of the data collection, represented essentially by :

- The existence of missing data relating to the medical treatment of victims who initially survived.

- Some results of toxicological and anatomopathological samples were missing

The strengths of our study were :
- The exhaustive nature of the sample, which can be considered representative of northern Tunisia (including all the governorates of northern Tunisia with the exception of Nabeul and Bizerte).

- The sample size was satisfactory.

2. Epidemiological study :

2.1. Prevalence of electrocutions :

In our study, the average rate of electrocution was 0.74/100,000 inhabitants. This rate was close to that of the study carried out in our department in 2017 (0.6/100,000 inhabitants)(9) and slightly lower than that observed in Kairouan in 2020 (0.94/100,000 inhabitants).
/100,000 inhabitants)(10). This finding was probably associated with the lack of compliance with workplace safety measures in central Tunisia compared with northern Tunisia. This rate was higher than in international studies: 0.53/100,000 inhabitants in Germany, 0.52 in Australia, 0.5 in the United States and 0.49 in Japan (12). This could be explained by the very young age at work in our population, non-compliance with or ignorance of general safety measures when handling electrical cables, and a lack of inspection and maintenance of electrical equipment.

2.2. Profile of victims :

2.2.1. Breakdown by age :

In our study, the average age of electrocutees was 39.68 with ranging from 8 months to 77 years of age. 47.6% of cases were aged between 18 and 39 years of age. Our results could be explained by the youth of the working population, as well as by the lack of professional experience of young people, which leads to higher risk behaviour in this age group. We found a second peak of 19% among victims aged between 50 and 60. This finding could be explained by the lack of vigilance and concentration among these victims, who were older and still working.Children were not spared in our study. They accounted for 5.6% of victims (seven cases). All were male. All the cases were accidental, and no cases of suicide by electrocution in children were found in our series. This rate was lower than that of the study carried out in Tunis in 2017 (9), which accounted for 13%. This could be explained by the fact that our study included only nine governorates in the north of Tunisia compared with ten in the other study. In Australia, children accounted for 11% of electrocution victims. The study concluded that children's easy access to faulty equipment in the domestic environment was the most common cause of electrocution. Older children are more likely to suffer accidental electrocution by adopting risky behaviour, or in work situations. The author also deduced that suicide by electrocution is a rare method of self-destruction in children. In fact, suicidal electrocution accounted for only 2% of all childhood suicides (13). The predominance of young age has also been noted in other Tunisian and foreign series, as illustrated in Table 17.

Table XVII: Breakdown by age group and studies

Place of	the study	Année de the study	Tranche affected	
Our study	Tunis	2024	39,68 18-39	
Studies Tunis(9)		2017	31,9	20-39
national	Kairouan(10)	2020	30	26-30
	Bangladesh(14)	2011	-	21-30
	China(15)	2010	31,77	-
	India(2)	2022	-	20-30
Studies	France (16)	2015	34	25-44
international	United States (17)	2014	35,2	25-34
	Sweden(18)	2006	38	-
	Bulgaria(19)	2010	35,25	-
	Quebec (20)	2001	35	-

2.2.2. Breakdown by gender :

According to our study, 90% of the victims were male. The predominance of males was noted in other national and international studies, as shown in Table 16. The predominance of men could be explained by the fact that men are more exposed to sources of electrical current than women (occupational accidents, domestic accidents linked to DIY activities and electrical maintenance, which are often carried out by men, and accidents on the public highway linked to risky behaviour, which is more marked in men)(21).

Table XVIII: Breakdown of victims by gender and education

	Year of the study	Men	Women
Our studyTunis	2024	90%	10%
Studies Tunis (9)	2017	88,1%	11,9%
nationalKairouan (10)	2020	91%	9%
Bangladesh (14)	2011	88,48%	11,52%
China (15)	2010	87,33%	12,67%
India (2)	2022	94,36%	5,63%
Studies Iran (22)	2006	94.6%	5,4%
internationalFrance (16)	2015	87%	13%
South Africa (23)	2018	82,1%	17,9%
Bulgaria (19)	2010	74.07%	25,93%
Quebec (20)	2001	96,77%	3,23%

2.2.3. Geographical breakdown :

According to our study, 71.4% of victims were of urban origin. This predominance was also observed in other Tunisian series. In fact, 88% of those electrocuted were of urban origin in the north of Tunisia in 2017 and 65% in Kairouan in 2020 [10,11]. This predominance has been noted in the literature, as described in the study carried out in Sweden in 2006, in South Africa in 2018 and in Canada in 2016 [24]. This finding could be explained by the high concentration of the industrial network and the use of increased use of domestic electrical appliances in urban areas (23),(18). However, a study in Bangladesh found that the mortality rate in rural areas was six times higher than in urban areas. According to the author, this reflects the rapid expansion of electrical connections and their increased use in rural areas(25).

2.2.4. Breakdown by victim's occupation :

In our series, the victims most affected were from the working class. This predominance has been noted in national studies: in Kairouan, 57.4% of victims were manual workers and electrical installation and maintenance workers, and in Tunis, in 2017, 74.3% of victims worked as manual workers, bricklayers or electricians. Internationally, a study in Turkey showed that most victims of occupational accidents were construction workers and electricians, with percentages of 21% and 19% respectively (21). Another study in Sweden showed that 46% of workers who died from electrocution were electricians (18). In the United States, and more specifically in Alabama, the occupational categories most affected by electrocution were electricians (18.5%) and manual workers (14.8%) (26).

According to these studies, what could encourage occupational electrical accidents is the increase in the number of hours worked, which leads to fatigue and a lack of caution. They also mention the lack of preventive measures on construction sites, the inexperience of seasonal workers, the large number of power tools used and the wear and tear on equipment in these occupations (18),(21),(26). A study in China revealed that welders, builders and decorators appeared to be more vulnerable to electrical injuries and had a higher number of fatalities. The author explained that this trend can be attributed to the fact that a greater number of workers carry out these occupations in less favourable conditions, often within small private companies (15).

2.3. Circumstances of electrocution :

2.3.1. Breakdown by season and month :

In accordance with national studies carried out in Tunis in 2017 (9) and in Kairouan in 2020 (10), the majority of electrocutions in our series occurred during the summer season (44%). The highest incidence rate was observed mainly in July and August with a percentage of 17.5% each.Internationally, the same results were found in Turkey (58% of electrocutions occurred in summer) (21), Bulgaria (60% of electrocutions) (27), India (33% of electrocutions) (28), (29) and the United States (29).United States (26). This finding was explained by the authors by: the increase in the number of constructions at this period (21),(26), the pressure to complete work before the winter season (work decreases due to weather conditions). Heat and longer working days may also be contributing factors (24). Studies have suggested that increased sweating in the summer reduces skin resistance, leading to an increase in the number of electrocutions(28),(29).

2.3.2. Breakdown by time of day :

According to our results, electrocutions occurred more frequently in the afternoon between 12pm and 6pm (45.2%). This peak was found in Kairouan (46.3%) (10). This could be explained by the lack of vigilance on the part of workers in the late morning and the increased use of electricity at this time of day. A study carried out in India found that all cases of electrocution were reported during working hours. According to the author, this shows that deaths due to electrocution are proportional to the use of electrical sources (29).

2.3.3. Breakdown by location of electrocution :

In our series, the majority of electrocutions occurred in the home. (46,8%). The rate of electrocution in the workplace was also high (34.1%). The place of electrocution varied significantly according to the occupation of the victims (p =0.000014). The two nationwide studies showed that electrocution was predominantly occupational (9),(10). These high rates of occupational accidents could be explained by negligent maintenance of equipment, lack of training and awareness of occupational safety, and failure to comply with safety instructions. Internationally, the results varied widely and differed from country to country. A study in Turkey found a predominance of electrocutions in the workplace with a percentage of 71%, the author linked this result to the acceleration of new construction sites and new industries in Turkey during this period. This acceleration was accompanied by a greater number of occupational accidents due to the absence of preventive measures for workers, most of whom were inexperienced (21).The maximum number of occupational electrocutions in our study occurred between the ages of 50 and 59 (11 cases). Indeed, advanced age could be considered a concentrating factor (30). All the women in our study were electrocuted at home. We found a significant relationship between the gender of the victim and the place of electrocution (p= 0.001). The extreme age ranges (<10 years and >69 years) were all electrocuted at home. A study carried out in India showed that 34.3% of fatal electrical injuries occurred in the home, and the majority of these accidents were caused by faulty household electrical appliances (28).

2.3.4. Breakdown by type of electric current :

High-voltage electrocutions were more common than low-voltage electrocutions in our series, with percentages of 52.5% and 47.6% respectively. The majority of low-voltage electrocutions occurred in the home in 68.3% of cases, whereas 60.5% of electrocutions occurring in the workplace were caused by high-voltage current. caused by a high-voltage current. We found a significant relationship between the type of current and the place of electrocution (p=0.00001). Furthermore, our study revealed a significant relationship between the type of current and the type of accident, highlighting a prevalence of domestic accidents involving low-voltage current, whereas accidents occurring in the workplace or in a public environment were more associated with high-voltage current (p=0.000008). Our results were similar to the Tunisian series. In fact, 63% of cases were linked to a high-voltage current in Tunis (9) and 66.7% of electrocutions in Kairouan (10). Internationally, studies have found divergent results. In South Africa, one study showed that low-voltage current was responsible for 72.2% of electrocutions (31). Another study in Turkey found that 61% of cases were caused by low-voltage current (21). A study in Croatia also found that electrocution by low-voltage current was predominant, with a rate of 75% (32). On the other hand, other series had found a predominance of electrocutions by high voltage current, such as the one carried out in India with a percentage reaching 56.11% (14), and the other in Canada with a rate of 72% (24).

2.3.5. Breakdown by causal agent :

The majority of electrocutions were caused by an exposed cable (64.3%). The remaining victims were electrocuted either by a faulty electrical appliance (24.6%) or by contact with an electrical socket (11.1%). The Tunisian studies did not specify the nature of the causal agent in their results.

On the other hand, international studies have identified the agent responsible for electrocution. An Australian study found that overhead power lines were the agent responsible for high-voltage electrocution. Contact with live wires during work, the use of extension cords with bare wires or defective electrical equipment, and the repair of electrical machines were the causes of death from low-voltage current (33). An Indian study showed that the main cause of electrocution was air coolers (4.0%), followed by bathroom fittings in the home (2.1%) and live bare wires in the workplace (4.4%). Electric water motors were also a frequent source of electrocution (3.7%), as were various other household electrical appliances and power poles. However, in around two-thirds of cases, the source was not mentioned in the report (34).

2.3.6. Distribution according to humidity conditions :

The majority of electrocutions occurred in a dry environment (71.4%). The study carried out in Tunis in 2017 found that electrocutions occurred in a damp atmosphere in 18% of cases. This atmosphere was mainly represented by: bath or shower (12%), wet hands (52%), wet floor (18%), wet hands and floor (4%), wet clothes (14%) (9). The study carried out in Kairouan showed a predominance of electrocutions in a damp environment (64.8%) (10). Internationally, a study in Australia found that all homicides and 23% of suicides were committed in a damp environment (emergence from an electrical appliance in a bath) (33). Another Canadian study found that 16% had reduced skin resistance due to damp extremities (20).In our study, we found that survival time varied significantly with humidity conditions (p=0.005). This is explained in the literature by the fact that skin resistance (which is the main barrier to electric current) is an important factor in determining current flow and that this resistance is influenced by skin humidity. It is therefore a factor that increases the risk of death by electrocution (33),(20)

2.4. Support :

2.4.1. Survival time :

The majority of victims died within the first 24 hours following electrocution (79.4%). Our results were consistent with Tunisian studies. Indeed, 64.9% of electrocution deaths in Tunis in 2017 and 74% in Kairouan had taken place on site (9) (10). This finding was similar in certain international series. However, a Canadian study found that 92% of electrocuted victims died at the scene or on arrival at hospital (20). A study in China found similar results. In fact, 92.96% died on arrival at hospital (15). This immediate death was explained in the literature by the fact that electrocution can lead to death by causing asystole, ventricular fibrillation or respiratory arrest, either by tetanic contraction of the respiratory muscles or by lesions affecting central respiratory control. However, death after 24 hours was related to other causes (20) (35) (36).On the other hand, other series had lower rates, such as the one carried out in Turkey, where the on-site death rate was 37.3% (35). We found a significant relationship between the type of current and survival time (p=0.0003). Almost all the victims electrocuted by a low-voltage current died within the first 24 hours (93.3%). This highlighted the severity of low-voltage electrification on the vital prognosis. A Chinese study linked this finding to the fact that low-voltage current could cause various cardiac anomalies, including heart rhythm disorders. High-voltage current, on the other hand, caused burns that do not usually result in immediate death (15).

2.4.2. Mode of delivery :

In our study, no victim was transported by the emergency medical service (SAMU). Only one victim was transported by non-medical means (by type B ambulance). The majority of victims were transported by the civil protection (83.3%). The study carried out in Kairouan found similar results. Only 9.3% of victims were transported by the SAMU and 11.1% by type B ambulance (10).According to the literature, the intervention of a medical team from the SAMU is indicated in all cases of electrification by a high-voltage current. Visit In the event of electrification due to a low-voltage current, the level of medical attention varies according to the symptoms observed. If the person presents a simple tremor without loss of consciousness, a quick consultation on the spot by a GP on duty is recommended. On the other hand, if a serious injury is suspected from the first call, the intervention of the Mobile Emergency and Resuscitation Service (SMUR) is systematic (36). Resuscitation must be carried out quickly, depending on the patient's condition. On the other hand, although the victim may appear to be dead, remarkable recoveries have been reported, so aggressive and prolonged resuscitation efforts must be undertaken (37). In Japan, they had even proposed the use of medical helicopters in cases of electrocution as a means of medical transport, as these victims were more likely to be successfully resuscitated (38).

3. Forensic study :

3.1. Thanatological findings :

3.1.1. Study of skin lesions :

3.1.1.1. Electrical brands :

Electrical marks are the only specific sign of the passage of electricity. They result from the heat produced by the electric current through the epidermis and dermis, a phenomenon known as the Joule effect, combined with metallisation due to the electrolytic release of metal ions from the electrode. They are mainly represented by the entry and exit points of the current. The entry point is characterised by a central area of mottled or whitish necrosis caused by arteriolar spasm, which is slightly depressed and hard to the touch, while the exit point is generally a small, well-defined area of white or grey necrosis, forming a small ulceration. In the event of exposure to high-voltage current, the ulceration may be more extensive. Sometimes these marks can be hidden by skin folds, hair, calluses on the hands, or by other types of skin burns such as those caused by an electric arc or clothing fire. The absence of electrical marks does not eliminate electrocution. According to the authors, this is due either to the low intensity of the current, or to the reduced resistance of the skin. by humidity or the extent of the skin surface in contact with the current (body emerged in water) (4), (12), (13), (39), (37).71.4% of the victims in our series had electrical marks. These marks were divided into an entry point in 34.1% of cases, an exit point in 7.9% and a combination of both entry and exit points in 29.4% of cases.National studies had found variable results in relation to the presence or absence of electric brands. Electric brands were found in only 47.6% of cases in Tunis and in 79.6% of cases in Kairouan (9,10). International studies, on the other hand, noted the presence of electric brands in the majority of cases. For example, in Turkey, electrical marks were found in 97% of cases (21). In India, an entry point was observed in 91.6% of cases (34). A study in Croatia found electrical marks in 79% of cases (32). A predominance of marks on the left upper limb (35.5%) was noted in our series. In 31% of cases, the portal of entry was in the left upper limb, whereas the portal of exit was more likely to be in the right lower limb (12.7%).Our study found the same findings as the international studies. However, in South Africa, marks on the upper limbs were more common than those on the lower limbs. In fact, 64% of cases showed lesions on the upper limbs (23). In Turkey, the portal of entry was located on the upper extremities in 74% of cases (21). Another study in the United States also found a predominance of upper limbs (5). The same result was observed in India, with the percentage of electrical marks on the upper extremities reaching 81.3% (6), (34). This finding could be explained by the fact that the victims most often came into contact with the source of the current either directly through their hands or through a conductive object they were holding. It is important for the examiner to trace the path of the electric current through the victim's body. This could give an idea of the degree of fatality of the current. According to the literature, it has been argued that the The most fatal current pathway involves contact with the right hand and exit through the feet, as this carries up to 8.5% of the total body current through the heart, as opposed to other pathways such as head to feet (up to 5.9%), left hand to feet (up to 5.1%), hand to hand (up to 4.4%) or foot to foot (up to 0.4%) (40).

3.1.1.2. Electrical burns :

Unlike thermal burns, the severity of electrical burns did not depend on the percentage of the skin surface burnt. In fact, electrical injuries are distinguished by the extent of internal damage that can lead to death, even though the area of skin affected may seem relatively small.It is common for deep burns to appear along the path of the current, particularly in the narrower, more resistant areas such as the limbs (41). In our series, severe electrical burns were present in 34.1% of cases, 67.4% of which were 3ème degrees. Nationally, all the victims of high-voltage current had burns with a skin surface area of burns varying between 1% and 99% per square metre and an average of 23% in Tunis (9). In Kairouan, 14.3% of victims had serious burns (10).A study in South Africa found that 73.6% of cases electrocuted by low-voltage current had no burns, 2.2% had 1er degree burns, 21.9% had second-degree burns and 1.1% had third-degree burns, while high-voltage current was responsible for 8.5% of second-degree burns, 62.8% of third-degree burns and 11.4% of fourth-degree burns. From this series, it would appear that deaths from high-voltage electrocution caused deeper burns than deaths from low-voltage electrocution (31). Another study in Croatia found extensive burns in 16% of cases (32). We found no other skin lesions. On the other hand, 4.8% of the victims had presented "crocodile skin" lesions, 3.2% had a vascular arborisation and 7.1% had carbonisation lesions. According to the literature, when an air gap forms between the conductor and the skin, the current can jump over this gap, causing a spark injury. This spark burn is caused by an extremely high temperature, leading to carbonisation of the keratin layer (12).
, (13). In the case of burns caused by high-voltage current, sparks can be generated over a distance of several centimetres. This can cause multiple lesions giving rise to a "crocodile skin" effect (40), (42). In Croatia, 4.5% of electrocuted victims showed charring following electrocution by a high-voltage current (32). In South Africa, the "crocodile skin" lesion was found in 1.1% of cases electrocuted by a low-voltage current and in 8.57% by a high-voltage current (31). It is sometimes possible to identify burn marks that reproduce the shape of the causal object. These marks could prove invaluable when the examiner sought to reconstruct events, and they could even reveal for the first time that death was caused by electricity, especially when the circumstances of the electrocution were unclear (40), (43). Sometimes, the forensic pathologist can diagnose electrocution through burns to clothing caused by the flame of the current as it leaves the human body, especially if the electrical marks are located in the folds of the skin, the hair or the calluses of the hands.

3.1.2. Asphyxia syndrome :

Our study found that the asphyxia syndrome was present in 75.4% of victims. It was mainly represented by pulmonary oedema in 75.4% of cases, followed by cerebral oedema (73%) and poly-visceral congestion (66.7%). Our results were similar to those of the study carried out in Tunis in 2017, which reported a high rate of non-specific asphyxia syndrome (82.2%) (9). This congestion of the internal organs was also observed in 92.1% of cases in a study in South Africa (23).

3.1.3. Associated trauma:

Associated trauma was found in more than a third of cases in our series (34.9%), of which 27.8% of cases had head trauma, 16.7% had chest trauma, 7.1% had abdominal trauma and 8.7% had polytrauma. These injuries were linked either to the victim falling from their own height or from a height, or to the victim being thrown following electrification. These findings highlighted the complexity of the traumatic injuries associated with electrocution deaths, which can make interpretation difficult in some cases. In view of their high frequency, it is crucial to pay particular attention to these injuries. National studies have also found a significant rate of trauma associated with electrocution. The study carried out in Tunis in 2017 found that electrocution was associated with trauma in 17.3% of cases. The study in Kairouan found that 37 % of victims had a trauma associated with electrocution (9), (10). Internationally, a study in Turkey found traumatic injuries in 30% of cases, and in 16% of cases, these injuries were related to a fall from a height following electrocution. The study found a significant relationship between the nature of the electric current and trauma. On the other hand, traumatic injuries were more frequent in accidents following electrocution by a high-voltage current (21). In South Africa, 37.1% of cases presented trauma associated with electrocution by a high-voltage current and 24.1% by a low-voltage current (31).

3.1.4. Additional post-mortem examinations :

3.1.4.1. Toxicological report :

In our series, a toxicological sample was taken in 45.2% of cases, and only one victim had a positive toxicological report with an assay of blood alcohol level of 0.69g/l. 8.7% of the cases had a negative toxicology report and the rest of the samples (35.7%) had not been recovered, which was a limitation of our study because it was not possible to make a true estimate of the rate of consumption of toxic substances at the time of the incident. In Kairouan, cannabis use was observed in 3.7% of cases. Alcohol was confirmed in only one case, with a blood alcohol level of 2.6 g/l, who was the victim of suicidal electrocution when he touched a high-voltage pole (10).In Croatia, alcohol concentrations were measured in 89.8% of cases. In 82% of these cases, the samples were negative for alcohol. All samples with positive alcohol concentrations (18%) were taken from male victims. Alcohol concentrations ranged from 0.53 g/kg in muscle tissue to 3.91 g/kg in blood and 5.81 g/kg in urine. No victims of professional electrocution and no minors tested positive for alcohol (32). In Sweden, alcohol was analysed in the blood and urine of 78% of victims electrocuted in the workplace. In 5% of cases, alcohol was detected in both blood and urine. Outside the workplace, 35% of victims tested positive for alcohol. 45.6% of them were riding in railway carriages at the time of the fatal accident. The majority of victims were aged between 15 and 29 (18).In Turkey, no traces of drugs were detected during toxicology tests. However, toxicological analyses revealed blood alcohol concentrations ranging from 8 to 84 mg/dl in 23% of cases. Of these, 17% were accidents at work. The author stated that alcohol consumption considerably reduces workers' attention span (21). The aim of these tests is to identify the circumstances behind cases of electrocution, particularly when they occur in the workplace. For example, a study carried out in the United States revealed that 69% of workers who suffered electrocution underwent toxicological tests. Of these, 22% tested positive for various substances, such ascannabis and alcohol (44).

3.1.4.2. Anatomopathological examination :

Histologically, it is difficult to make a formal distinction between electrical burns and burns of other origins, particularly thermal. This is because the epidermal lining can detach and rise up to form a bubble, creating a large space underneath. The cells of the epidermis are often elongated, with the nuclei of the lower layers oriented and stretched horizontally; this was initially explained by an electromagnetic effect, but a similar appearance can be observed in purely thermal burns (40).

According to a study carried out in France, It is true that the stretching of the nuclei, the basophilic coloration of the epidermis and the homogenisation of the dermis are secondary consequences of the thermal effect. However, the combination of intra- and sub-epidermal vacuolisation seems suggestive of an electrical burn. Good lateral limitation of the lesions is also an argument in favour of electrical burns (45).

Electron microscopy can reveal various changes, particularly in the nuclei of skin cells, which appear distorted with clumped chromatin. Janssen grouped together a range of electrical histological lesions in his work on forensic histology, but it seems clear that few features are absolutely specific to electrical burns compared with classic thermal burns (40), (46).

On the other hand, the presence of metallisation on the skin (as a result of a physical process that causes the metal conductors to melt) is specific to electrical burns and indicates direct contact with an electrical source (12), (45). Among the techniques used to detect metallisation, energy dispersive X-ray spectroscopy stands out for its high sensitivity (capable of detecting even a few micrograms of the metallic element), its non-destructive nature, its speed of execution and its ability to perform a multi-element analysis (12). In terms of the heart, we can find a series of lesions that are similar to consists of: aggregates of cardiomyocytes sometimes showing hyper-contraction and sometimes distension with enlargement or rupture of the intercalary discs, non-eosinophilic bands corresponding to hyper-contracted sarcomeres alternating with zones of separation of hyper-stretched sarcomeres. These changes appear to be characteristic of ventricular fibrillation, although they are not specific to electrocution. The detection of lesions suggestive of ventricular fibrillation on anatomopathological examination, combined with the information gathered during the investigation, led to the conclusion that cardiac arrest was due to ventricular fibrillation induced by electrocution (45).Our study found that a pathological examination was carried out in 9.5% of cases. Only two results were obtained. The first involved a skin fragment and showed epidermal changes consistent with a burn. The second sample concerned organ fragments and showed, in the heart: a focal dense eosinophilic appearance of myocardial cells without neutrophils, indicating acute cellular suffering; in the lungs: recent focal alveolar haemorrhage with no other abnormalities apart from moderate non-inflammatory oedema. The congestive brain, cerebellum, trunk, pancreatic, renal and splenic tissues were without significant abnormalities.In Kairouan, histological examination was carried out in 14.8% of victims and in 13% of cases this examination was in favour of electrocution (10). In addition, a study in Turkey found that in 8.1% of cases, there was no histopathological change that could be attributed to the electric current, while the other cases showed histological findings in favour of electrocution (35).

3.1.5. Mechanism of death :

The most frequent fatal process is cardiac arrhythmia, generally ventricular fibrillation ending in asystole. The current has a profound effect directly on the myocardial syncytium, which can cause dislocation of the conduction pathways. Less frequently, if a current passes through the thorax and abdomen, it can cause respiratory paralysis due to spasms of the intercostal muscles and diaphragm. The electric current can also travel through the head and neck. This could have a direct impact on the brain stem, leading to paralysis of the cardiac or respiratory centres (40).

In Kairouan, ventricular fibrillation was observed in 16.7% of cases at the time of initial assessment, and only one case presented with a circumferential myocardial infarction at autopsy (10).In our study, the investigations carried out in the emergency department were not available. However, we can deduce that the final mechanism of death was a cardiac or respiratory cause related to electrocution in 68.3% of cases, given the presence of electrical marks and the observation of an isolated asphyxic syndrome with visceral congestion without extensive burns or associated serious trauma. 91.7% of victims electrocuted by a low-voltage current died as a result of isolated electrocution, and therefore probably as a result of arrhythmia or respiratory paralysis.In the case of high-voltage electrocution, these cardio-respiratory mechanisms could contribute to the fatal outcome, but the mechanism most frequently encountered was extensive burns to the body, with the infectious and hypovolaemic complications they could cause (42). In our study, we found that in 19.8% of cases, death was secondary to septic shock complicating extensive, deep and superinfected electrical burns. 88% of these victims had been electrocuted by a high-voltage current.

It is important to note that injuries associated with electrocution are more common in industrial accidents and work on power lines. Victims of shock may be thrown from a height or suffer intense muscle spasms that can lead to fractures and other serious injuries (40). However, in our study 11.9% of cases had a serious trauma associated with electrocution resulting in death. 86.7% of these victims were electrocuted by a high-voltage current. According to our study, the mechanism of death varied significantly according to the type of electric current (p=0.00005).

3.2. Forensic form :

3.2.1. Accidental form :

The accidental form was the most frequent in our series (97.6% of cases). It was divided into four types: 47.6% of victims were electrocuted following a domestic accident, 34.1% following an accident at work, 14.3% following a road traffic accident and 1.6% of cases were electrocuted during a copper theft. Our results were in line with national studies. The accidental form accounted for 92.6% in Kairouan and 99% in Tunis(9), (10). The same findings were observed internationally. For example, the rate of fatal electrical accidents was 98.7% in South Africa (23), 100% in Maharashtra in India (29), 99% in Turkey (21), 100% in the United States (21) and 100% in Australia (22).in china (15) and 69% in Australia (33).In Tunisia, compensation for accidents at work and occupational illnesses is governed by Law No. 94-28 of 21 February 1994 for the private sector and Law No. 95-56 of 28 June 1995 for the state sector. An accident at work is defined by Article 3 of these two laws: "An accident at work is deemed to be, regardless of the cause or place of occurrence, any accident occurring as a result of or in the course of work, to any worker in the service of one or more employers. An accident occurring to a worker while travelling between his place of work and his place of residence is also deemed to be an accident at work, provided that the journey has not been interrupted or diverted for a reason dictated by his personal interest or unrelated to his professional activity" (47), (48). The victim or the victim's beneficiaries must inform the employer of the accident on the same day or within 48 working hours at the latest. In the private sector, the employer must report the accident to the CNAM (Caisse Nationale d'Assurance Maladie) within 3 working days of being notified. A copy of the declaration must be forwarded to the nearest police or national guard station and to the Labour Inspectorate. The employer must provide the victim with a medical certificate so that he can seek treatment. In the state sector, the employer must report the accident to the Central Medical Commission at the Prime Ministry within 3 working days of being notified. A copy of the declaration must be sent to the CNRPS (Caisse Nationale de la Retraite et de Protection Sociale). Under article 45 of law no. 94-28 of 21 February 1994, in the event of death as a result of an accident at work in the private sector, the victim's spouse and children or, failing that, ascendants and descendants are entitled to a death pension. Article 49 of the same law also specifies the method for calculating the pension. In the public sector, compensation is the same as that provided for the private sector, with a few differences specified in law no. 95-56 of 28 June 1995 (48). These differences mainly concern the formulas for calculating the pension. A Spanish study announced that accidents at work represent a major problem in contemporary economic structures. However, when these accidents result in the loss of human life, the associated economic and social cost becomes even more worrying. Although the development of prevention policies, both at governmental and sectoral level, has contributed to a gradual reduction in accidents at work, the number of fatal accidents remains high (49).

In our study, occupational accidents accounted for more than a third of electrocutions (34.1% of cases). This high rate points to a failure in occupational safety measures, and therefore calls for the application of preventive measures to reduce this scourge. We are going to discuss a particular case of road accidents related to copper theft.

Special case: Copper thieves :

We recorded 2 cases of electrocution following the theft of copper. The victims were males aged between 22 and 38. They had no occupation and were of low socio-economic status. The memorabilia reported the theft of copper metals by the victims. deceased. The last contact with the victims was at night, and they would be found deceased near a power pole. One case presented burn lesions on the gloves he was wearing. Burn lesions compatible with electrical marks were noted on the right hand. Craniofacial and thoracic trauma were found in both cases. Abdomino-pelvic and axial trauma were found in only one case. Electricity has become a target for two types of theft: theft of service and theft of equipment. Copper is the most widely used metal because of its remarkable electrical conductivity and malleability, which enables it to carry high currents in industrial installations and electrical distribution cabinets (50). Because of its high market value, thefts of objects made from this metal seem to have been on the increase for some time, leading to a rise in high-voltage electrical accidents and premature deaths from electrocution (50). The victims were generally young, male and of low socio-economic status. The profile of our cases was consistent with that described in the literature (31),(50). Electrical marks were mainly found on the dominant limb. Burns caused by high-voltage current predominated on all four limbs, particularly the hands and interdigital spaces. Associated trauma was frequent, often related to high projections. The combination of craniofacial and thoracic trauma was the most frequent, as described in the literature (6),(50),(31).

3.2.2. Suicide :

After the January 2011 revolution, suicide rates rose to significant levels in northern Tunisia, with an increase of 26%, becoming a major public health problem. The methods most frequently used to commit suicide over the past decade have been hanging, self-immolation and self-poisoning (51). Cases of suicide by electrocution are relatively rare and have not been sufficiently studied in our country. In our series, the forensic form was suicidal in only three cases. victims (2.4% of cases). The three victims were male, aged between 28 and 35. They were single with low socio-economic status. Two victims had a psychiatric history. The three suicidal acts were committed on the public highway by climbing an electricity pole. They were all caused by a high-voltage current. One victim died on the spot. The other two were hospitalised more than 24 hours before their deaths.National and international studies have reported the same findings in relation to the low rate of electrical suicides (9) (10).(15) (21) (23) (29) (32) (33). In contrast to our study, a study in Australia found that 48% of suicides by electrocution occurred in people aged over 60. The study found two distinct groups of victims of suicidal electrocution. The first group consisted mainly of elderly men with technical skills in electricity, who committed suicide by plugging themselves directly into an electrical socket. The second group, made up mainly of women, included individuals who electrocuted themselves in a water bath using an electrical appliance. This study found that many of them suffered from multiple physical and psychological comorbidities (52). A study in Bulgaria found that suicides by electrification accounted for 6.24% of all electrocutions. The average age of the victims was 45.1 years, ranging from 14 to 75 years. Men (91.5%) clearly outnumbered women (8.5%). Children under 18 accounted for a relatively small proportion (3.4%). As for the type of electrical current used, 42.4% of victims chose low voltage. The most preferred method of electrical suicide involved contact between the victim and an electric cable, accounting for 47.4% of cases. Climbing and contact with a high-voltage power line accounted for a further 13.6%. In third place, cases of climbing a pole and contact with a live wire from a street power line accounted for 11.64%(53).

4. Preventive measures :

4.1. Primary prevention :

4.1.1. At home:

Domestic electrifications generally occurred in the paediatric population when children, often of pre-school age, inserted a conductive object into an electrical socket, either by inserting their fingers, touching or carrying a bare wire or an extension cord connected to the current, or by making contact with a faulty appliance (54). A French study suggested a number of simple measures to avoid electrification:

- Protect the wall sockets.
- Protect electrical wires.
- Remove any bare wires.
- Unplug all electrical appliances after use.
- Do not leave extension leads connected to the mains plug lying around.
- Avoid placing electrical appliances near water (bath, bathroom).
- Ban mobile heaters in bathrooms.

This study pointed out that active prevention, which involves educating families about the risks and installing protective systems, had not proved effective in reducing domestic accidents (54). On the other hand, a study in South Africa demonstrated the effectiveness of systematic preventive home visits in improving the compliance of electrical installations (55). In France, new homes would have to comply with the NF C 15-100 standard, which guaranteed, among other things, that each dwelling would have a general electrical control and protection system, including circuit breakers and fuses to prevent overcurrents, as well as differential devices to detect current leaks. In addition, the would require the installation of wall sockets fitted with shutters.For older homes, it is recommended that you use safety sockets with shutters. It is also advisable to upgrade the electrical installation, replace faulty sockets and repair bare wires. Since 1 January 2009, it has been compulsory to carry out a safety diagnosis of the electrical installation for homes over 15 years old, in accordance with Decree 2008-384 of 22 April 2008. The responsibility for carrying out the necessary work lies with the homeowner (54).

4.1.2. At work :

Occupational accidents are a major issue throughout the world. More than 350,000 deaths were recorded in 2001. Around 1,000 people lose their lives every day as a result of accidents at work. The number of accidents at work resulting in at least three days' absence from work in 2001 is estimated at nearly 270 million (56).

In northern Tunisia, electrocution was the third leading cause of traumatic death in the workplace, accounting for 18.5% (57).

In order to prevent accidents at work, the causes must be detected initially:

- Dangerous behaviour: overconfidence, working haphazardly, carelessness and disregard for operating procedures, lack of concentration and lack of knowledge or experience,

- Dangerous conditions: faulty appliances, dangerous equipment, a shortage of safety supplies and a lack of instructions for carrying out tasks, work carried out very close to overhead power lines or the construction of unauthorised buildings.
- Uncontrollable events: storms, earthquakes, floods. Before starting any work, all safety measures must be in place. rigorously put in place, and no work should start without a detailed plan for safe and complete operation.

An Indian analysis revealed the crucial importance of creating well-detailed procedures and data sheets and adhering to them to avoid catastrophic results (58). A structured approach is therefore essential:

- Identify the specific nature of the tasks to be carried out.
- Carefully assess the risks associated with each task.
- Implementing risk reduction techniques.
- Develop mitigation strategies to limit hazards.
- Anticipate scenarios where the situation could worsen.
- Give priority to establishing a safe working environment.
- Take preventive measures to prevent incidents.
- Set up a warning and communication system in the event of loss of control.

- Carry out thorough checks before starting each task.
- Integrate an instant safety system to remind people of the importance of using safety equipment and complying with procedures.

- Adapt professional electrical equipment to the recommended safety parameters.

- Department workers need relief bars to work on reception lines

- If workers do not use safety devices, a means of locking the system must be devised.

By following these steps, it is possible to effectively reduce the risk of accidents and promote a safe working environment (58).

Individuals with no technical training were associated with a disproportionate number of accidents, which supports the idea that it is necessary for workers receive training to guard against electrical hazards, in particular by learning how to disconnect sources of electricity quickly (59). It is crucial to assign a specific task to each individual to ensure safe and efficient execution. The diversity of mental tasks can compromise concentration on the task in hand, increasing the risk of errors.

4.2. Secondary prevention :

It is essential that witnesses of an electrification accident give priority to their own safety to avoid the risk of over-accident. Before handling the victim, it is important to ensure that contact with the conductive agent and the electrical source has been eliminated. Once the injured person has been isolated and protected, the first step in the emergency chain is to contact the medical emergency service on the free number 190. The regulating doctor adapts the emergency response by activating the appropriate technical services at the same time as sending in the emergency medical services.Calling civil protection on number 198 in the event of an electric shock is a common mistake in our Community. Civil protection is a non-medical means of transport, so transporting an electrification victim is beyond its remit.According to a French study, all cases of electrification by high-voltage current require the intervention of a SAMU medical team. The level of medical assistance required varies according to the symptoms described in the event of a domestic electric shock. If there is an isolated tremor, with no loss of consciousness and mild symptoms, it is recommended that a GP on duty at the scene should be consulted quickly. If there is an abnormality in the electrocardiogram, medical transport to a cardiological monitoring service is then recommended. On the other hand, if there is a suspicion that an important function has been impaired as soon as the initial alarm is raised, it is essential to intervene immediately with the SMUR (36).

4.3. Tertiary prevention :

Treatment of burns caused by high-voltage current requires complicated surgical procedures, often involving amputations in around 37% of cases. Local progression is manifested by the formation of fibrous scar tissue with electrophysiological dysfunction (39). We will discuss the main sequelae after electrification and the therapeutic means available for better social and professional reintegration.

4.3.1. Neurological sequelae :

Peripheral neuropathy is the most common form of damage, with paresthesia and neuropathic pain. Most cases are reversible and sensitive to analgesic treatments such as tricyclic antidepressants and anticonvulsants(60).

4.3.2. Orthopaedic sequelae :

Fitting orthopaedic devices to amputated limbs and rehabilitation remain the therapeutic solutions available, even if they are only partially effective. Indeed, the predominance of proximal joint involvement makes fitting difficult. In addition, fibrosis corresponding to the current pathway is frequently the site of chronic infection, and a source of delayed healing and therefore delayed rehabilitation (39).

4.3.3. Psychiatric sequelae :

Depressive syndrome, severe neurotic or psychotic disorders, as well as minor manifestations such as amnesia, all associated with the concept of "post-traumatic syndrome" have been reported in the literature (39),(60). The importance of early psychological care, maintained throughout the rehabilitation and reintegration period, is crucial in positively influencing long-term outcomes (61).

CONCLUSIONS

Electricity is widely used in everyday life, which increases the risk of electrical trauma, a very serious event that can lead to significant morbidity and mortality. Electrifications were particularly serious because of the high rates of immediate death of the victims or following complications caused by poly-visceral failure, whether or not linked to trauma or extensive burns. Electrocution is a violent death, which requires the medical-legal obstacle to burial to be stated on the medical death certificate in order to initiate legal proceedings. It is difficult to make this diagnosis in the absence of a witness, because of the not inconsiderable rate of electrocutions with no anomalies on examination of the body. The aim of our study was to describe the epidemiological profile and lesion characteristics of the bodies of victims of electrocution in the north of Tunisia, to identify the circumstances in which electrocutions occur and to suggest ways of improving the prevention and management of victims of electrocution.We carried out a descriptive study with retrospective data collection over a four-year period from 1[er] January 2019 to 31 December 2022 in the Forensic Medicine Department of Charles Nicolle Hospital in Tunis, covering all cases of death by electrocution whose body had undergone a medico-legal autopsy. We included all cadavers autopsied at the forensic medicine department of Charles Nicolle Hospital whose autopsy concluded that they had been electrocuted. We did not include all the cases of corpses autopsied in the forensic medicine department of the Charles Nicolle Hospital in Tunis whose cause of death was other than electrocution. Similarly, cases of Fulguration (electrification by lightning) were not included in our study. We excluded corpses in a state of advanced putrefaction and decomposition. The data was collected from the registers of the forensic medicine department and the forensic medical files, each containing a judicial requisition and a copy of the forensic autopsy report. The data collected was entered and analysed using SPSS 23 (Statistics Package for the Social Science). Figures and tables were produced using Microsoft Excel 2013.At the end of this study, we recorded 126 victims of electrocution, with an average rate in relation to the general population of 0.74/100,000 inhabitants and 1.4% in relation to the thanatological activity of our department. There was a clear male predominance (90%), with an average age of 39.68. The age groups most affected were those between 26 and 39 (47.6%), with extremes ranging from 8 months to 77 years. Electrocution mainly affected blue-collar workers (61.1% of cases). Electrocutions were more frequent between midday and 6pm (45.2%), on Saturdays (19%), during the summer season (44%) and in the Greater Tunis region (80.1%). Most of these were accidents (97.6%), of which 47.6% were domestic accidents, 34.1% accidents at work, 14.3% accidents on the public highway and 1.6% related to attempted copper theft. We found a significant relationship between the gender of the victim and the place of electrocution (p=0.001). High-voltage electrocutions accounted for 52.5% of cases, with a stripped cable as the main causal agent in 64.3% of situations. The majority of deaths (79.4%) occurred within the first 24 hours, without EMS intervention, and 62.7% of victims died at the scene, without medical assistance. In terms of injuries, an electrical mark was observed in 71.4% of cases, with 29.4% of victims presenting both an entry and an exit site. The upper limbs were most frequently affected as entry points for electric shocks, while the lower limbs were more often affected as exit points. Associated traumatic lesions were observed in 34.9% of cases. In most cases, toxicological and anatomopathological analyses were not carried out, which was a limitation of our study. According to our study, the profile of the victims corresponded to those mentioned in the national and international scientific literature, with mainly male victims working as manual labourers in the following sectors construction or industry. Our work has also highlighted the crucial importance of pre-hospital medical care and the shortcomings of intensive care in our country.Our results had highlighted the need to reinforce the training of primary care physicians on the specific lesion characteristics of electroshocks, given their crucial role in the reporting of electrical incidents in the workplace. Their involvement is also essential in the early treatment of electroshock victims in order to reduce the mortality rate. Identifying the forensic form of electrocution is not always straightforward for the forensic pathologist. Some cases of accidental electrocution may in fact conceal homicide. This is why in-depth investigations, as well as additional toxicological and anatomopathological examinations, are essential to establish with certainty the forensic nature of these cases. Likewise, it is essential to have information on the most common circumstances of occurrence and the victimology profile most often observed, so that front-line doctors can consider raising the medico-legal obstacle to burial if this diagnosis is suspected, and so that the forensic pathologist can take this diagnosis into account during the assessment even in the absence of electrical marks or thanatological signs in favour.

REFERENCES

1. De Carolis J, La Rose A. Annual energy outlook 2023 release at resources for the future. [On line]. Mar 2023 [Accessed 25 Mar 2024]; [25 pages]. Available from: URL: [cited 13 Feb 2024]. Available from:
https://www.eia.gov/outlooks/aeo/pdf/AEO2023_Release_Presentation.pdf

2. Shobhana S, Raviraj K. Pattern of electrocution deaths autopsied in South India a16 year retrospective study. J Forensic Med. 2022 Jun;13(1):1-7.

3. Champy P, Eteve C, Durand Prinborgne C, Hassenforder J, De Singly F. Dictionnaire encyclopédique de l'éducation et de la formation. 2ème edition. Paris: Nathan; 2000. 1167.

4. Shaha KK, Joe AE. Electrocution-related mortality: a retrospective review of 118 deaths in Coimbatore, India, between january 2002 and december 2006. Med SciLaw. 2010 Apr;50(2):72-4.

5. Arnoldo BD, Purdue GF, Kowalske K, Helm PA, Burris A, Hunt JL. Electrical injuries:a 20-year review. J Burn Care Rehabil. 2004 Nov;25(6):479-84.

6. Kumar S, Verma AK, Singh US. Electrocution-related mortality in northern India a5-year retrospective study. Egypt J Forensic Sci. 2014 Mar;4(1):1-6.

7. Eidgenössisches Starkstrominspektorat. Swiss Federal Inspectorate for Heavy Current Installations ESTI. [Online]. Nov 2022 [Accessed 25 March 2024]; [30 pages] .
the URL:

https://www.esti.admin.ch/inhalte/user_upload/ESTI_Taetigkeitsbericht_2 022_E R.pdf

8. Owona Manga LJ, Kouassi Yao M. Étude des accidents électriques d'origineprofessionnelle à Yaoundé. Ann Burns Fire Disasters. June 2017;30(2):91-4.

9. Jendoubi S. Les électrocutions au nord de la Tunisie étude sur 10 ans (2005-2014) [thesis: medicine]. Tunis: University of Tunis El Manar; 2017.

10. Jemli I. Aspects médico-légaux des électrocutions dans la région de kairouan àpropos de 54 cas [thesis: medicine]. Sousse: University of Sousse; 2020.

11. Institut National de la Statistique. Inflation rate. [On line]. Apr 2024 [Accessed 25 March 2024]. Available at URL: https://www.ins.tn/

12. Bellini E, Gambassi G, Nucci G, Benvenuti M, Landi G, Gabbrielli M, et al. Death by electrocution: histological technique for copper detection on the electric mark. Forensic Sci Int. 2016 Jul;264:24-7.

13. Byard R, Hanson K, Gilbert J, James R, Nadeau J, Blackbourne B, et al. Death due to electrocution in childhood and early adolescence. J Paediatr Child Health. 2003Jan;39(1):46-8.

14. Akber EB, Haque ST, Sultana S, Barua AK, Hossain Z, Jahan I. Jurisprudential analysis of death due to electrocution. Cent Med Coll J. 2022 Jun;5(1):13-9.

15. Liu S, Yu Y, Huang Q, Luo B, Liao X. Electrocution-related mortality: a review of 71 deaths by low-voltage electrical current in Guangdong, China, 2001-2010. AmJ Forensic Med Pathol. 2014 Sep;35(3):193-6.

16. Institut de Veille Sanitaire. Electrocutions électrisations en France métropolitaine.enquête permanente sur les accidents de la vie courante (EPAC, 2004-2011). [Online]. Mar 2015 [Accessed 25 March 2024]; [6 pages]. Available from URL:
file:///C:/Users/DELL/Downloads/TR15L112+(e%CC%81lectrocution+Cepi Dc197

9_2011+Epac2004_2011).pdf

17. Zhao D, Thabet W, McCoy A, Kleiner B. Electrical deaths in the US construction: an analysis of fatality investigations. Int J Inj Contr Saf Promot. 2014 Sep;21(3):278-88.

18. Lindström R, Bylund PO, Eriksson A. Accidental deaths caused by electricity in Sweden, 1975-2000. J Forensic Sci. 2006 Nov;51(6):1383-8.

19. Dokov W. Electrocution-related mortality: a review of 351 deaths by low- voltage electrical current. Ulus Travma Acil Cerrahi Derg. 2010 Mar;16(2):139-43.

20. Bailey B, Forget S, Gaudreault P. Prevalence of potential risk factors in victims of electrocution. Forensic Sci Int. 2001 Nov;123(1):58-62.

21. Akçan R, Karacaoglu E, Keten A, Odaba□i AB, Kanburoglu Ç, Tümer AR, et al. Electrical fatalities in Ankara over 11 years. Turk J Med Sci. 2012 Jan;42(3):533-8.

22. Sheikhazadi A, Kiani M, Ghadyani MH. Electrocution-related mortality: a survey of 295 deaths in Tehran, Iran between 2002 and 2006. Am J Forensic Med Pathol. 2010 Mar;31(1):42-5.

23. Von Caues S, Herbst CI, Wadee SA. A retrospective review of fatal electrocution cases at tygerberg forensic pathology services, Cape Town, South Africa, over the5-year period 1 january 2008 - 31 december 2012. S Afr Med J. 2018 Nov;108(12):1042-5.

24. Kim H, Lewko J, Garritano E, Sharma B, Moody J, Colantonio A. Construction fatality due to electrical contact in Ontario, Canada, 1997- 2007. Work. 2016 Jun;54(3):639-46.

25. Shawon RA, Ferdoush J, Ali AH, Biswas A, Rahman AF, Mashreky SR. Alarming rise in fatal electrocutions in Bangladesh: comparison of two national surveys. Burns. 2019 Sep;45(6):1471-6.

26. Taylor AJ, McGwin G, Davis GG, Brissie RM, Rue LW. Occupational electrocutions in Jefferson County, Alabama. Occup Med. 2002 Mar;52(2):102-6.

27. Dokov W. Assessment of risk factors for death in electrical injury. Burns. 2009 Feb;35(1):114-7.

28. Behera C, Sikary AK, Rautji R, Gupta SK. Electrocution deaths reported in South Delhi, India: a retrospective analysis of 16 years of data from 2002 to 2017. Med Sci Law. 2019 Oct;59(4):240-6.

29. Mukherjee B, Farooqui JM, Farooqui AJ. Retrospective study of fatal electrocution in a rural region of western Maharashtra, India. J Forensic Leg Med. 2015 May;32:1-3.

30. Tchicaya AF, Aka IA, Gafarou Touré AA, Nguessan MA, Guiégui CP, Kouassi YM, et al. Analysis of electrical accidents among employees of an electrical power distribution company in Togo. Arch Mal Prof. Feb 2020;81(1):24-31.

31. Blumenthal R. A retrospective descriptive study of electrocution deaths in Gauteng,South Africa: 2001-2004. Burns. 2009 Sep;35(6):888-94.

32. Kuhtic I, Bakovic M, Mayer D, Strinovic D, Petrovecki V. Electrical mark in electrocution deaths a 20-years study. Open Forensic Sci J. 2012 Jan;5(1):23-7.

33. Wick R, Gilbert JD, Simpson E, Byard RW. Fatal electrocution in adults a 30-year study. Med Sci Law. 2006 Apr;46(2):166-72.

34. Behera C, Sikary AK, Rautji R, Gupta SK. Electrocution deaths reported in South Delhi, India: a retrospective analysis of 16 years of data from 2002 to 2017. Med Sci Law. 2019 Oct;59(4):240-6.

35. Akçan R, Hilal A, Gülmen M, Çekin N. Childhood deaths due to electrocution in Adana, Turkey. Acta Paediatr. 2007 Mar;96(3):443-5.

36. Bertin Maghit M, Mazaud A, Spann C, Fayolle Pivot L, Quang DL, Rimmelé T, et al. Management of the electrified or struck by lightning patient. [On line]. Mar 2015 [Accessed on 25 March 2024]; [18 pages].   Available from

URL:https://sofia.medicalistes.fr/spip/IMG/pdf/prise-en-charge- du-patient-electrise- ou-foudroye-39-bertin-maghit-1442329293.pdf

37. Leibovici D, Shemer J, Shapira SC. Electrical injuries: current concepts. Injury. 1995 Nov;26(9):623-7.

38. Ishikawa K, Jitsuiki K, Ohsaka H, Yoshizawa T, Obinata M, Omori K, et al. Management of a mass casualty event caused by electrocution using doctor helicopters. Air Med J. 2016 May;35(3):180-2.

39. Gueugniaud PY, Vaudelin G, Bertin-Maghit M, Petit P. Accidents d'électrisation. [On line]. Oct 1997 [Accessed 25 March 2024]; [20 pages]. Available at à the URL: https://urgences- server.fr/IMG/pdf/electrisation.pdf

40. Saukko P, Knight B. Knight's forensic pathology. 4th Edition. London: CRC Press; 2015.

41. Jowdar S, Kismoune H, Boudjemia F, Bacha D. Electrical burns, retrospective and analytical study of 588 cases over a decade 1984-1993. AnnBurns Fire Disasters. Mar 1997;10:20-7.

42. Byard RW. Electrocution post-mortem presentations, problems and pitfalls. Forensic Sci Med Pathol. 2023 Mar;19(1):91-3.

43. Bux R, Amendt J, Rothschild MA. A fatal search for worms a peculiar electrical accident. Leg Med. 2003 Dec;5(4):242-5.

44. Ramirez M, Bedford R, Sullivan R, Anthony T, Kraemer J, Faine B, et al. Toxicologytesting in fatally injured workers: a review of five years of Iowa FACE cases. Int JEnviron Res Public Health. 2013 Nov;10(11):6154-68.

45. Franchet C, Savall F, Guilbeau Frugier C, Dedouit F, Telmon N, Delisle MB, et al. Electrocutions: contribution of anatomopathological examination. A propos of two cases.Rev Med Leg. May 2013;4(2):97-102.

46. Janssen W. Forensic histopathology. New York: Springer-Verlag; 1984.

47. Republic of Tunisia. Law n° 94-28 of 21 February 1994, on the compensation of damages resulting from accidents at work and occupational diseases (J.O.22February 1994).Available at : http://chaexpert.com/documents/Loi%2094-28%20Accidents%20of%20work%20and%20Occupational%20Diseases.pdf

48. Republic of Tunisia. Law no. 95-56 of 28 June 1995 on the special compensation scheme for injuries resulting from accidents at work and occupational diseases in the public sector. (J.O. 4 July 1995). Available: http://www.atds.org.tn/LOI1995.pdf

49. Fuentes Bargues JL, Sánchez Lite A, González Gaya C, Artacho Ramírez MA. Descriptive analysis and a proposal for a predictive model of fatal occupational accidents in Spain. Heliyon. 2023 Nov;9(11):e22219.

50. Taylor AJ, McGwin G, Brissie RM, Rue LW, Davis GG. Death during theft from electric utilities. Am J Forensic Med Pathol. 2003 Jun;24(2):173-6.

51. Ben Khelil M, Gharbaoui M, Farhani F, Zaafrane M, Harzallah H, Allouche M, et al.Impact of the Tunisian revolution on homicide and suicide rates in Tunisia. Int J Public Health. 2016 Dec;61(9):995-1002.

52. Chan P, Duflou J. Suicidal electrocution in Sydney a 10- year case review. J ForensicSci. 2008 Mar;53(2):455-9.

53. Dokov W. Forensic characteristics of suicide by electrocution in Bulgaria. J ForensicSci. 2009 May;54(3):669-71.

54. Claudet I, Maréchal C, Debuisson C, Salanne S. Risk of rhythm disorders and domestic current electrification. Arch Pediatr. Apr 2010;17(4):343-9.

55. Odendaal W, Van Niekerk A, Jordaan E, Seedat M. The impact of a home visitation programme on household hazards associated with unintentional childhood injuries: a randomised controlled trial. Accid Anal Prev. 2009 Jan;41(1):183-90.

56. Hämäläinen P. The effect of globalization on occupational accidents. Saf Sci. Juil 2009;47(6):733-42.

57. Ben Khelil M, Harzallah H, Elmoulehy Majed H, Belghith M, Hamdoun M. Workplace traumatic accidental death in Northen Tunisia. Tunis Med. 2019 Jul;97(7):918-24.

58. Rathour JH, Sinha DR. Proactive measures to prevent accidents due to electrocution from recurrence. J Res Adm. 2024 Jan;6(1):1278-89.

59. Edlich RF, Farinholt HA, Winters KL, Britt LD, Long WB. Modern concepts of treatment and prevention of electrical burns. J Long Term Eff Med Implants. 2005Dec;15(5):511-32.

60. Wilbourn A. Peripheral nerve disorders in electrical and lightning injuries. Semin Neurol. 1995 Sep;15(3):241-55.

61. Primeau M, Engelstatter G, Bares K. Behavioral consequences of lightning and electrical injury. Semin Neurol. 1995 Sep;15(3):279-85.

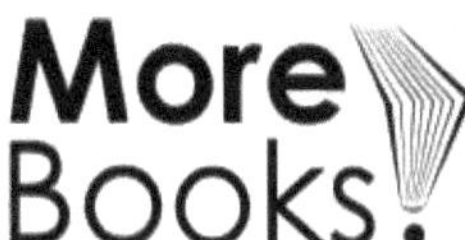

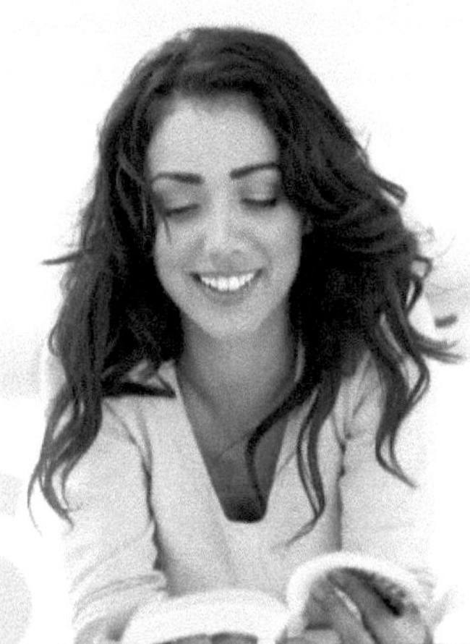

yes I want morebooks!

Buy your books fast and straightforward online - at one of world's fastest growing online book stores! Environmentally sound due to Print-on-Demand technologies.

Buy your books online at
www.morebooks.shop

Kaufen Sie Ihre Bücher schnell und unkompliziert online – auf einer der am schnellsten wachsenden Buchhandelsplattformen weltweit! Dank Print-On-Demand umwelt- und ressourcenschonend produziert.

Bücher schneller online kaufen
www.morebooks.shop

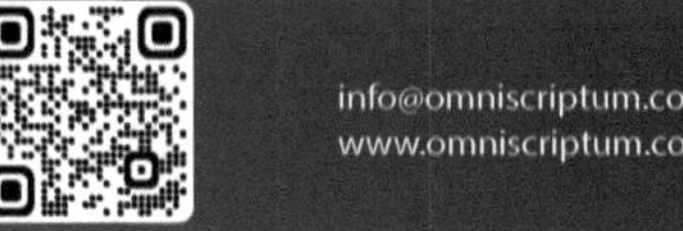

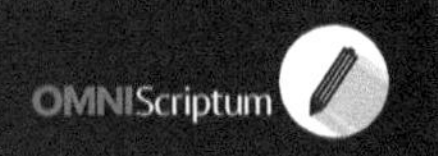

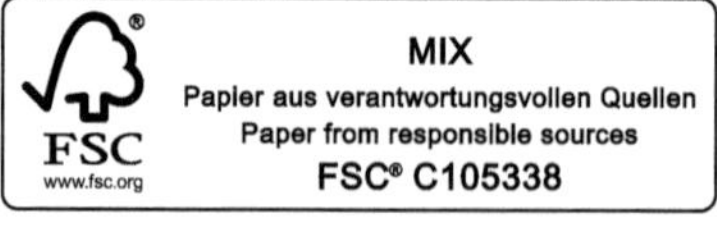

Printed by Books on Demand GmbH, Norderstedt / Germany